# Oral mucositis

W0043035

Development of this book was supported by funding from Helsinn

# Oral mucositis

**Stephen T Sonis**
Division of Oral Medicine and Dentistry
Brigham and Women's Hospital
Boston, Massachusetts
USA

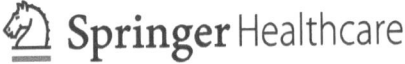

Published by Springer Healthcare Ltd, 236 Gray's Inn Road, London, WC1X 8HB, UK.

www.springerhealthcare.com

© 2012 Springer Healthcare, a part of Springer Science+Business Media.

British Library Cataloguing-in-Publication Data.

A catalogue record for this book is available from the British Library.

ISBN 978-1-908517-63-0

Project editor: Tamsin Curtis
Designer: Joe Harvey
Artworker: Sissan Mollerfors
Production: Marina Maher
Printed in xxx by xxx

# Contents

# Author biography

**Stephen T. Sonis,** DMD, DMSc received his DMD from Tufts University, and then entered a combined doctorate and clinical specialty training program at Harvard University. Following completion of his degree and residency, he was awarded a Knox Fellowship to study tumor immunology at Oxford University, UK. He returned to the United States to accept joint positions at the Peter Bent Brigham Hospital, Sidney Farber Cancer Center, and the Harvard School of Dental Medicine.

Dr Sonis' research converged on studies to define the biology and clinical significance of cancer regimen-related mucosal toxicities. The results of his studies on the molecular and cellular pathogenesis of mucositis have established the basis of a mechanistic paradigm for epithelial injury, and have provided treatment targets for biological and pharmaceutical development. Recognizing that genetics play a role in patient risk for mucositis and other toxicities, Dr Sonis and his collaborators have identified specific canonical pathways that are critical in toxicity development and have used these to form the basis for models of gene-based risk prediction. With the application of network theory to cancer-related toxicities, Dr Sonis and his colleagues have built on earlier work to define specific toxicity constellations in patients receiving chemotherapy. Dr Sonis has broad experience in clinical trial design, implementation, and endpoint quality management. Many of his former students and residents now hold academic and clinical leadership positions.

Dr Sonis has published extensively on the clinical, biological, and health economic aspects of cancer and complications associated with its treatment. He is the author of over 200 original publications, reviews and chapters, 7 books, and 5 patents. He has lectured extensively on the clinical and biological aspects of cancer regimen-related toxicities and cancer diagnostics. Dr Sonis serves on a number of editorial boards, and is a founding member of the International Society of Oral Oncology and the International Academy of Oral Oncology.

# Chapter 1

# Introduction

Since Madame Curie discovered radium in 1897 and the application of radiation to treat of cancers in the days before World War I, injury to the mucosal surfaces of the mouth (oral mucositis or OM) has been a prominent toxicity of antitumor therapies. With the advent of chemotherapy in the late 1940s, the etiology of mucositis broadened. Despite its extended clinical legacy, it is only within the past decade or so that mucositis' complex pathobiology has become fully appreciated. One thing that remained consistent from the initial descriptions of its clinical manifestations has been the frustration on the part of clinicians and patients with the scarcity of therapeutic options to prevent or treat the condition, or effectively ameliorate its symptoms.

## Nomenclature

Historically, oral mucosal injury associated with cancer treatment was referred to as "stomatitis". However, because "stomatitis" was also used to refer to many oral mucosal conditions with etiologies exclusive of cancer treatment-related damage (eg, infection), a more specific term was needed. Consequently the term "mucositis" was recognized as being more appropriate for lesions specifically associated with cytotoxic cancer therapy, and in 2007 was adopted and assigned an ICD-9 code of 528.0. The ICD-10 code for OM is K12.3.

S. T. Sonis, *Oral Mucositis*,
DOI: 10.1007/978-1-907673-46-7_1, © Springer Healthcare 2012

## Clinical presentation

In its most advanced clinical form, OM presents as confluent, deep, and devastatingly painful ulcerations of the oral mucosa. However, like most diseases, mucositis has a clinical continuum. At its beginning stages or in its most mild form, mucositis presents as mucosal erythema (Figure 1.1) and is accompanied by a feeling of burning, not dissimilar to that which results from a severe hot food burn. In some patients who receive selected chemotherapy regimens for the treatment of solid tumors (eg, breast or colorectal cancers), mucositis may not progress to more severe mucosal changes.

In contrast, many patients go on to develop the more severe and classic forms of mucositis, which is characterized by ulcerative lesions. The ulcers of mucositis tend to be deeper and markedly more painful than those typically associated with canker sores (aphthous stomatitis) or traumatic lesions. Unlike aphthous stomatitis (Figure 1.2), mucositis ulcers do not have a typical inflammatory component and so do not have a peripheral ring of erythema. Ulcer development is associated with increased pain and an inability to tolerate normal foods. It is not unusual for patients with significant mucositis to exclude solid foods completely. Ulcers may be focal and localized or consolidated and diffuse. Their borders are generally poorly defined.

There are no sentinel sites for lesions of mucositis. Any part of the movable mucosa can be involved, although the buccal mucosa (cheeks) (Figures 1.3 and 1.4), floor of the mouth, lateral and ventral borders of the tongue (Figure 1.5), and soft palate are most frequently involved. Interestingly, the more heavily keratinized mucosa is usually not involved in mucositis. Thus in cancer patients with ulcerative lesions of the hard palate, dorsal surface of the tongue, and gingiva, an etiology other than mucositis should be suspected. Most common lesions in these areas are the consequence of viral (herpes simplex) or fungal (candidiasis) etiology (Chapter 8).

## The course of mucositis

The course of mucositis is generally predictable and depends on the cancer treatment associated with its generation.

## Early mucosal changes following the initiation of radiation therapy

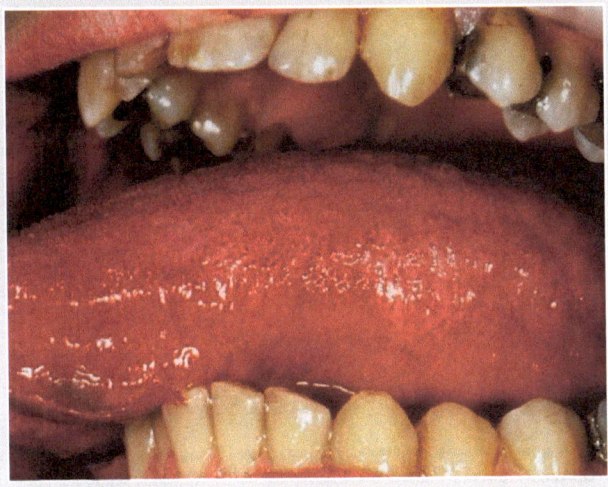

**Figure 1.1 Early mucosal changes following the initiation of radiation therapy.** The left lateral border of the tongue is mildly erythematous and edematous.

## An aphthous lesion of the labial mucosa

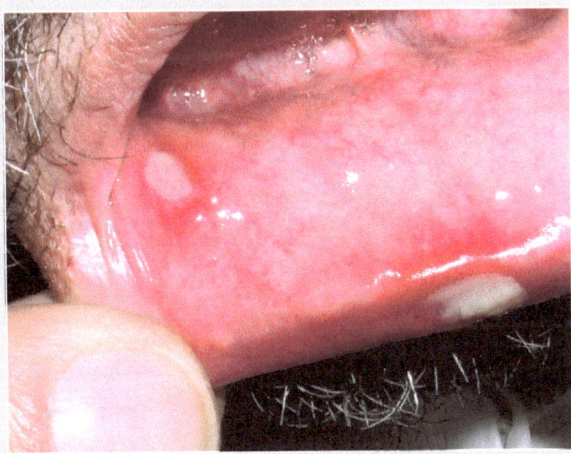

**Figure 1.2 An aphthous lesion of the labial mucosa.** Note that the ulcer is round, with a grayish necrotic center, and surrounded by an erythematous ring. Despite the fact that the lesion is shallow, it still elicits discomfort. In contrast to lesions of mucositis, aphthous lesions are discrete and recurrent.

Ulcerative mucositis of the cheek in a patient being treated with radiation therapy for oral cancer

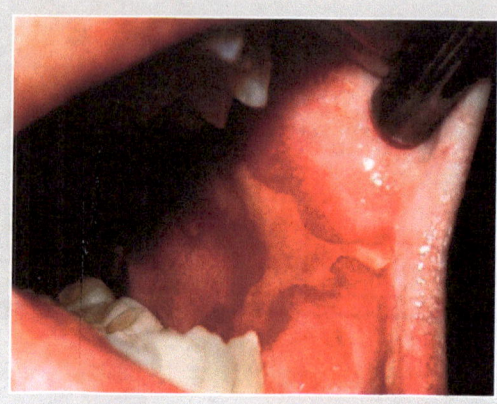

**Figure 1.3 Ulcerative mucositis of the cheek in a patient being treated with radiation therapy for oral cancer.** The ulcerative area of the lesion is covered by a graying pseudomembrane and surrounded by erythema. The surrounding mucosa is infected. Although the figure is limited to the buccal mucosa, lesions were extensive, bilateral, and involved the soft palate. © Nathaniel Treister, reproduced with permission.

Oral mucositis involving the buccal mucosa

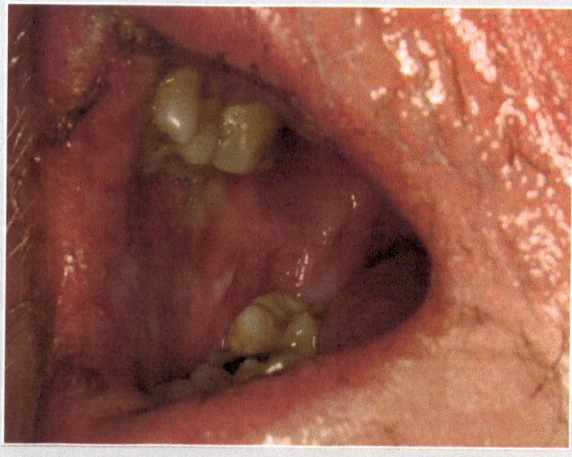

**Figure 1.4 Oral mucositis involving the buccal mucosa.** This patient presents with ulcerative mucositis of the right buccal mucosa, which developed during his chemoradiation therapy for the treatment of head and neck cancer. Areas of ulceration, possibly exacerbated by tooth trauma, are visible.

Oral mucositis involving the ventral surface of the tongue

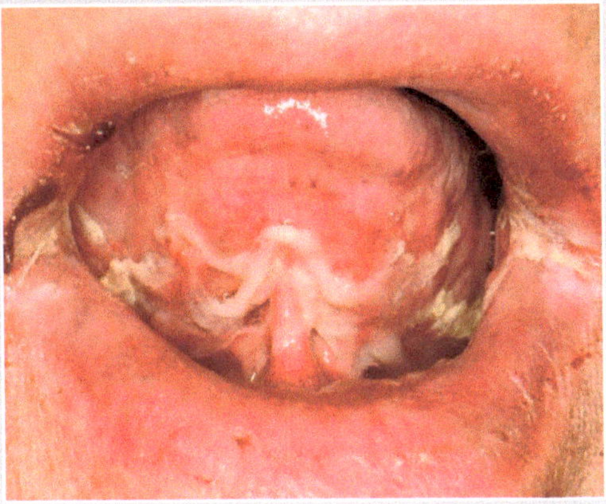

**Figure 1.5 Oral mucositis involving the ventral surface of the tongue.** Mucositis is often associated with conditioning regimens for hematopoietic stem cell transplant. In this case, the patient developed severe mucositis. Here, the ventral surface of the tongue can be seen to have marked ulceration and pseudomembrane formation. Bilateral involvement of the buccal mucosa and floor of the mouth were also present. © Nathaniel Treister, reproduced with permission.

## Mucositis induced by chemotherapy

For patients being treated with chemotherapy, the first signs of mucositis usually begin about 3 to 4 days after infusion with a feeling of mucosal irritation, which is accompanied by ulcer development.. This is also true of patients receiving conditioning regimens in preparation for hematopoietic stem cell transplants (HSCT). Mucositis tends to increase in intensity to peak 3–5 days later and persists for another 3–5 days (Figure 1.6).

## Mucositis induced by radiotherapy

In contrast, mucositis induced by radiation therapy is less acute both in its onset and resolution. Among patients with cancers of the head and neck, radiation is typically administered in fractionated daily doses of 2 Gy given Monday through Friday and continuing until a total dose of 60 Gy to 70 Gy has been given. Thus patients are planned to receive a total of 10 Gy per week. The majority of patients also receive concomitant chemotherapy. Typical regimens include cisplatin given either weekly or thrice during radiation treatment (days 1, 21, and 42). Chemotherapy

Mucositis of the left buccal mucosa

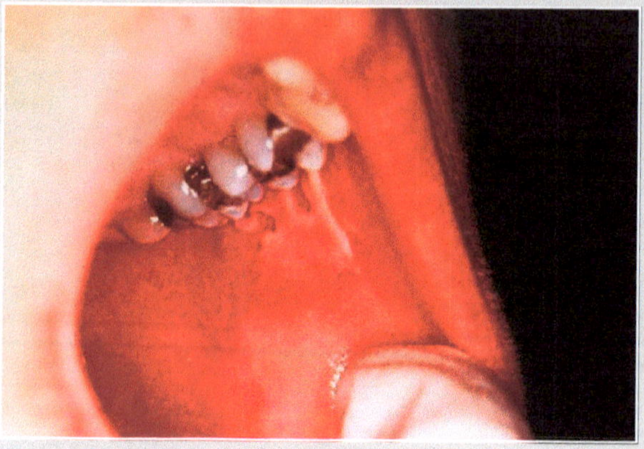

**Figure 1.6 Mucositis of the left buccal mucosa.** Pseudomembrane formation and erythema are clearly seen in this patient who has late stage mucositis. In the majority of cases mucositis resolves spontaneously. © Nathaniel Treister, reproduced with permission.

in these cases functions as a radiosensitizer. Patients begin to develop mucosal soreness by the end of week 1. The intensity of mucositis builds until ulceration occurs, in most cases by the end of week 2, and then consolidates to form confluent mucosal ulcers by the end of the third week. Since treatment is ongoing, patients can expect to have persistent ulcerative mucositis until 2–4 weeks after their last dose of radiation. In most cases, ulcers spontaneously resolve without scarring.

Development of this book was supported by funding from Helsinn

# Chapter 2

# The pathobiology of oral mucositis

## Historical concepts

Our understanding of the pathogenesis of OM has matured markedly over the past decade. Prior to the late 1990s the prevailing mechanism by which mucositis occurred focused on direct but nonspecific cell death mediated by either chemotherapy or radiation (Figure 2.1) [1]. The concept was simple: since neither chemotherapy nor radiation could differentiate between rapidly dividing (and DNA synthesizing) tumor cells or the rapidly dividing cells of the basal epithelium, these normal "mother" cells were killed, and replenishment of the normally renewing epithelium was eliminated. As a result, the story went, the mucosa would become atrophic and, if there was no replacement of the epithelium, ulceration developed. Ulcers would become secondarily colonized with bacteria, run their course, and then, if there were no extenuating circumstances, go on to spontaneously heal.

Increasing interest in mucositis spurred more in depth studies of its biology primarily as a way to develop targets for treatment.

## Biologically complex etiology of mucositis

In the late 1990s a series of studies was published in which the pathobiology of mucositis was studied in animal models that closely duplicated the human condition [2,3]. The results of these studies revealed findings which, when viewed comprehensively, led to a completely new hypothesis about how mucositis occurs and strongly suggested that the initial damage

S. T. Sonis, *Oral Mucositis*,
DOI: 10.1007/978-1-907673-46-7_2, © Springer Healthcare 2012

**Simple model of mucositis development due to chemotherapy- or radiation-mediated cell death**

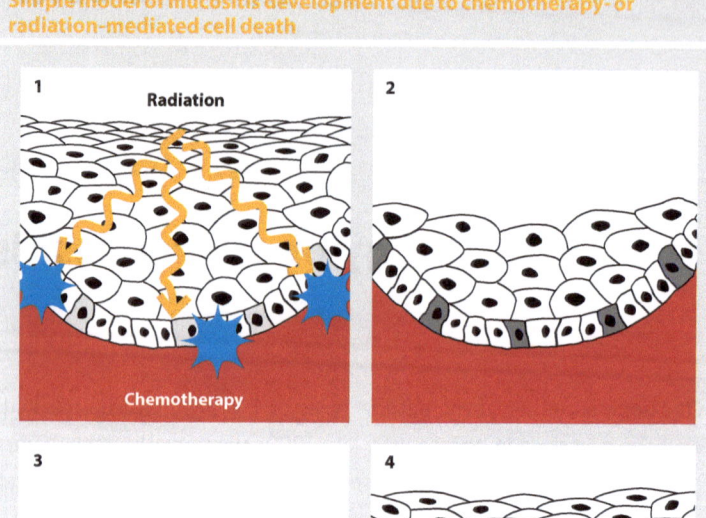

**Figure 2.1 Simple model of mucositis development due to chemotherapy- or radiation-mediated cell death.** Historically, mucosal injury was attributed to the direct effects of radiation and chemotherapy on epithelial stem cells of the mucosa. It was suggested that clonogenic cell death eliminated the renewal capacity of the epithelium. As a consequence the tissue became atrophic and then ulcerated. Subsequent studies have shown that the pathogenesis is much more complex.

takes place in the cells and tissues of the submucosa. This injury leads to the generation of signaling pathways that ultimately target the cells of the basal epithelium and leads to their demise. Since the first description of this new hypothesis, supporting data has been obtained from numerous studies [4]. These results confirm the concept that mucositis results from the cumulative impact of a number of biological pathways that originate in the submucosa and ultimately target the oral epithelium. These have been summarized in a five-stage schema (Figure 2.2) [5].

## Stage 1 – Initiation

The initiation phase is characterized by direct DNA injury caused by radiation or chemotherapy and subsequent strand breaks that result in clonogenic death of basal epithelial cells. Even more significant from the standpoint of ultimate tissue damage is the generation of reactive oxygen species (ROS) [6]. It has been recently suggested that cells damaged by chemotherapy and radiation may release endogenous damage-associated pattern molecules (CRAMPs), which then bind to specific receptors and contribute to the initiation of stage 2 [7].

## Stage 2 – Primary damage response

Chemotherapy, radiation, ROS, and CRAMPs initiate a series of cascading and interacting biological events, including the activation of a number of transcription factors, such as nuclear factor Kappa-B (NF-κB), Wnt, p53, and their associated canonical pathways [4].

Of the many canonical pathways that contribute to the development of mucositis, the NF-κB pathway is one of the best studied and provides an excellent example of the complexity of the process leading to ulceration. Chemotherapy and radiation can directly activate NF-κB. Indirectly, it can be activated by ROS or by receptor-bound CRAMPs. As a result, up to 200 genes may be expressed. Among these are genes associated with the production of molecules, which have demonstrated activity in the pathogenesis of mucositis including proinflammatory cytokines and cytokine modulators, stress responders (eg, COX-2, inducible NO-synthase, superoxide dismutase), and cell adhesion molecules. Furthermore, cell death (via apoptosis) may occur following NF-κB activation [8].

Other pathways have also been identified as playing significant roles in regimen-related mucosal injuries. Among the most significant are those associated with nitrogen metabolism, Toll-like receptor signaling, B-cell-receptor signaling, P13K/AKT signaling and mitogen-activated protein kinase (MAPK) signaling, to name a few [4,9]. In addition, other radiation- and chemotherapy-induced mucosal damage is associated with the ceramide pathway and fibrinolysis and the stimulation of matrix metalloproteinases (MMPs) [4,9].

## A multiple mechanism model for the pathobiology of mucositis

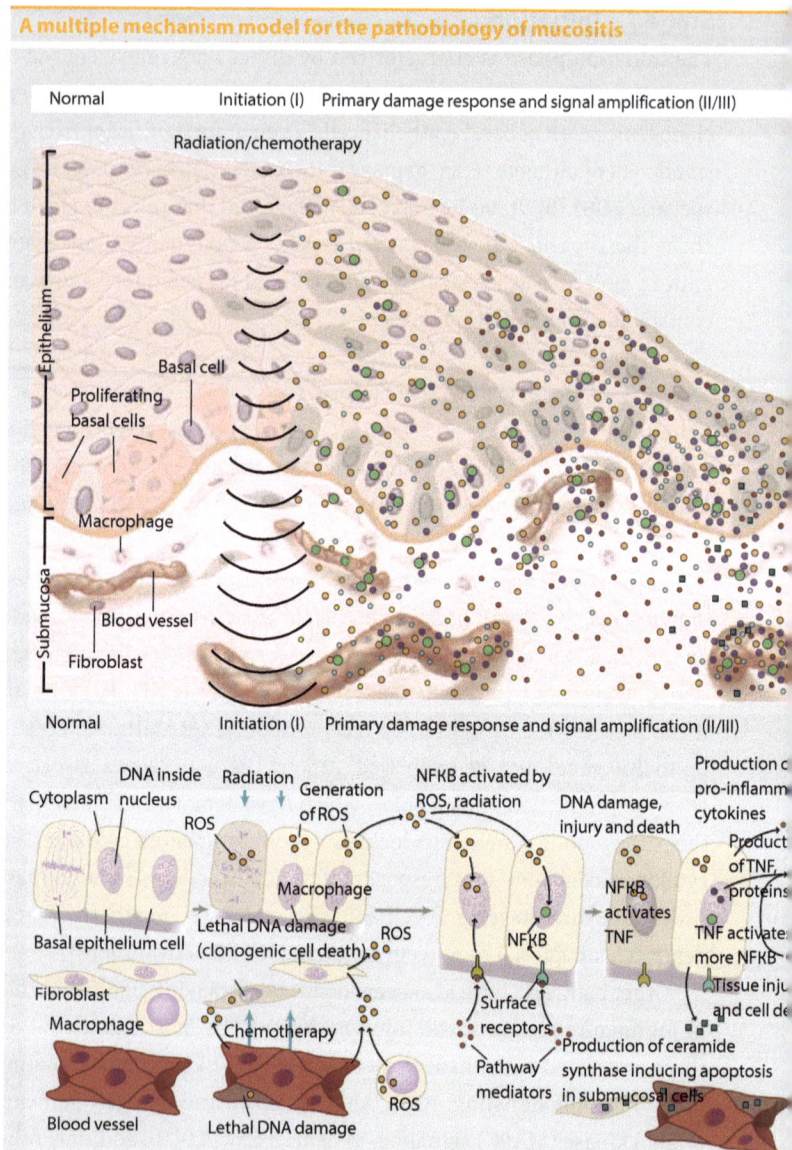

**Figure 2.2 A multiple mechanism model for the pathobiology of mucositis.** The pathobiology of mucositis as a five stage process. The key biological processes associated with the pathogenesis of oral mucositis can be arbitrarily divided into five stages: initiation, the primary damage response (messaging and signaling), amplification, ulceration, and healing. Reproduced with permission from Sonis [5].

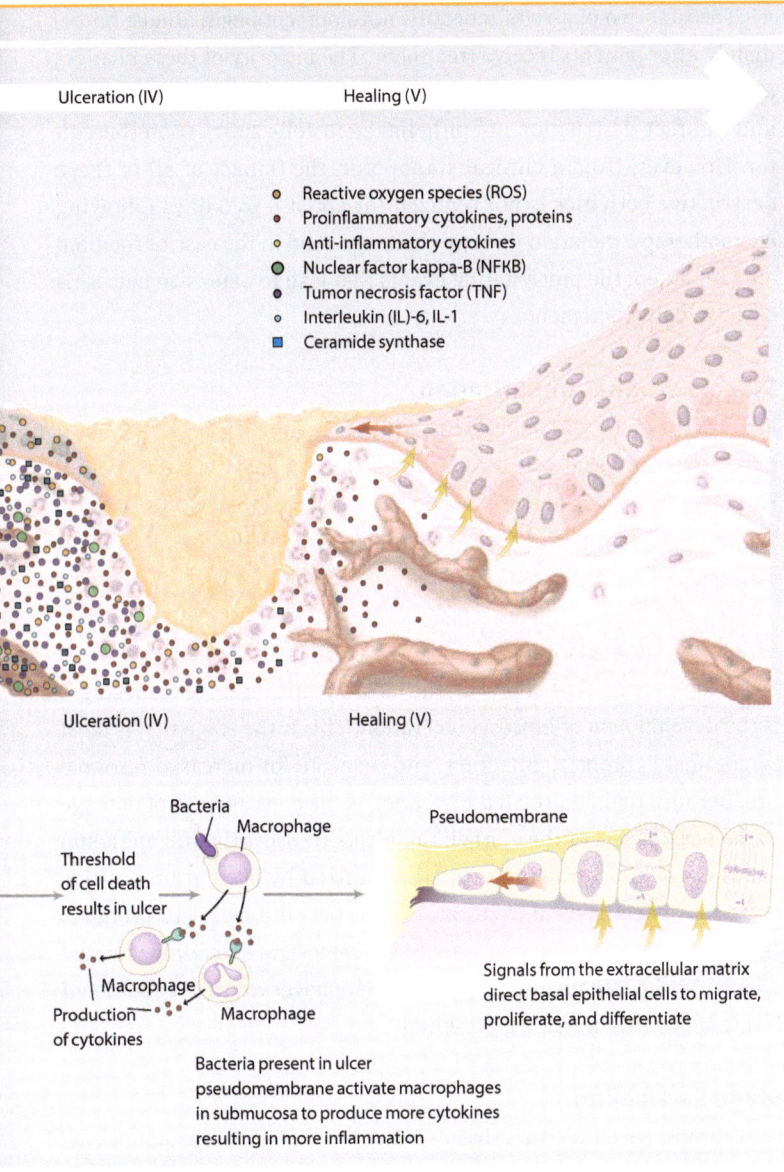

Ulceration (IV)    Healing (V)

- Reactive oxygen species (ROS)
- Proinflammatory cytokines, proteins
- Anti-inflammatory cytokines
- Nuclear factor kappa-B (NFKB)
- Tumor necrosis factor (TNF)
- Interleukin (IL)-6, IL-1
- Ceramide synthase

Ulceration (IV)    Healing (V)

Bacteria
Macrophage

Pseudomembrane

Threshold
of cell death
results in ulcer

Macrophage

Production
of cytokines    Macrophage

Signals from the extracellular matrix
direct basal epithelial cells to migrate,
proliferate, and differentiate

Bacteria present in ulcer
pseudomembrane activate macrophages
in submucosa to produce more cytokines
resulting in more inflammation

The first two phases of mucositis development begin almost immediately after patients receive treatment. The majority of these changes are seen within the cells and tissues of the submucosa and both direct and indirect destruction of epithelial stem cells starts soon thereafter. However, from a clinical standpoint, the impact of all of these destructive activities is not realized for about 4 to 5 days following chemotherapy/radiation therapy challenge. And in the case of fractionated radiation, the precipitating events that lead to extensive mucositis occur in daily increments.

## Stage 3 – Signal amplification

Many of the molecules induced by the primary response have the ability to positively or negatively feedback and alter the local tissue response. For example, tumor necrosis factor (TNF) may positively feedback on NF-κB to amplify its response, and initiate MAPK signaling, leading to activation of Jun N-terminal kinase (JNK) signaling [5].

## Stage 4 – Ulceration

For the patient and the clinician, the most significant stage of mucositis is the development of mucosal ulceration. This is the stage that is most symptomatic, prone to infection, and requisite for increased resource use. Because regimen-related ulceration is the consequence of damage at the basal layers of the epithelium, ulcers transect the full epithelial thickness. Once formed, ulcers are colonized by both gram positive and gram negative oral bacteria, which spew out cell wall products (see Figure 3.6) [4]. These molecules are capable of extending mucosal damage as they stimulate infiltrating macrophages to release additional levels of pro-inflammatory cytokines.

## Stage 5 – Healing

For the most part, the ulcerative lesions of mucositis heal spontaneously, although this too is the result of a series of biological signals originating in the submucosa [4,6]. Signaling molecules from the extracellular matrix direct the migration, proliferation, and differentiation of the epithelium bordering ulcerative areas. The epithelium extends beneath surface debris, fibrin, and cells to restore the mucosa's continuity [4,6].

# References

1 Lockhart PB, Sonis ST. Relationship of oral complications to peripheral blood leukocyte and platelet counts in patients receiving cancer chemotherapy. *Oral Surg Oral Med Oral Pathol.* 1979;48:21-28.

2 Sonis ST, Tracy C, Shklar G, et al. An animal model for mucositis induced by cancer chemotherapy. *Oral Surg Oral Med Oral Pathol.* 1990;69:437-443.

3 Sonis ST, Edwards L, Lucey C. The biological basis for the attenuation of mucositis. The example of interleukin-11. *Leukemia.* 1999;13:831-834.

4 Sonis ST. Mucositis: The impact, biology and therapeutic opportunities of oral mucositis. *Oral Oncol.* 2009;45:1015-1020.

5 Sonis ST. Pathobiology of oral mucositis: novel insights and opportunities. *J Support Oncol.* 2007; 5(9 suppl 4):3-11.

6 Sonis ST. A biological approach to mucositis. *J Support Oncol.* 2004;2:21-32.

7 Sonis ST. New thoughts on the initiation of mucositis. *Oral Dis.* 2010;16:597-600.

8 Sonis ST. The biologic role for nuclear factor-kappaB in disease and its potential involvement in mucosal injury associated with anti-neoplastic therapy. *Crit Rev Oral Biol Med.* 2002;13:380-389.

9 Sonis ST. The pathobiology of mucositis. *Nat Rev Cancer.* 2004;4:277-284.

Development of this book was supported by funding from Helsinn

# Chapter 3

# The epidemiology and risk assessment of mucositis

## Epidemiology

OM is among the most common and dreaded toxicities of cancer therapy [1]. It occurs in almost all patients who receive radiation therapy in which areas of the oral or oropharyngeal mucosa are included in the treatment field. Thus for patients with cancers of the mouth, oropharynx, hypopharynx, larynx, nasopharynx, and salivary glands, clinically significant OM occurs in about 70% of patients [2].

Recipients of conditioning regimens in preparation for HSCT are also considered to be in an especially high risk group for OM [3]. Aside from patient-associated risk factors (see below), the stomatotoxicity of individual conditioning regimens impact OM frequency and severity. For example, the incidence of severe (WHO grade ≥3) OM among patients with multiple myeloma or non-Hodgkin's lymphoma receiving conditioning regimens of high dose melphalan or carmustine, etoposide, cytarabine, and melphalan (BEAM), was reported to be 46% and 42% respectively [4]. In contrast, 98% of patients with hematological malignancies who received a conditioning regimen consisting of cyclophosphamide, etoposide, and total body irradiation developed severe OM [5].

### Inconsistencies in reporting oral mucositis

While there is reasonable clarity around the frequency of OM in patients in the categories discussed above, there is wide discrepancy in its incidence in patients with the most common tumor types: breast, colorectal,

S. T. Sonis, *Oral Mucositis*,
DOI: 10.1007/978-1-907673-46-7_3, © Springer Healthcare 2012

and lung cancers. In general, the incidence of mucositis in these patients has been underreported (Figure 3.1) [6].

Among the most common regimens for breast cancer (ie, AC+T – doxorubicin, cyclophosphamide, and paclitaxel or docetaxel), ulcerative mucositis occurs in about 20% of patients during the first cycle of treatment. If that group of patients receives the same dose of the same drugs in a second cycle, the frequency of OM jumps to 70% [7]. Interestingly, some of the newer regimens for metastatic breast cancer are even more stomatotoxic. The incidence of OM is more than 60% in patients receiving docetaxel and capecitabine, with 15% of patients developing severe OM [8].

There is rarely more inconsistency in the reporting of OM than among patients being treated with the standard 5-fluorouracil- (5-FU) containing regimens for colorectal cancer (CRC). The literature suggests that ulcerative OM occurs with a frequency of somewhere between 15% and 28% in patients receiving the most common 5-FU-based regimens [9]. Yet in a recent study, over 70% of CRC patients noted significant mouth and throat soreness following their treatment [10]. Furthermore, it appears that women are more likely to develop OM in response to 5-FU than men [11]. The reason for this difference has not been defined.

Newer drugs and regimens vary in their stomatotoxicity. Nineteen percent of elderly patients at risk of myelodysplastic syndrome were noted to have ulcerative OM in response to oral clofarabine [12]. In contrast, 70% of patients receiving pralatrexate developed mucositis, with 21% noted to have severe forms of OM [13]. The use of the novel

**Reasons for under-reporting of mucositis**

Among patients receiving multiple cycles of treatment, toxicity reporting may be limited to the first cycle only

Cited or mentioned toxicities associated with a regimen may be limited to only grades considered to be severe (3, 4)

Toxicity scales are not uniform in assessment criteria. Consequently a severe grade in one scale may not be severe in another (see Chapter 6)

The uniformity with which clinicians assess the mouth varies widely

Figure 3.1 Reasons for under-reporting of mucositis.

microtubule inhibitor vinflunine resulted in about 20% of nonsmall cell lung cancer patients developing OM [14].

Mammalian target of rapamycin inhibitors have been approved for the treatment of renal carcinomas and are being investigated as therapy for other cancer types including sarcoma. Mucosal ulcerations are among the most common toxicities (about 40%) associated with this drug class [15] and are even higher when combination regimens are used. For example, 60% of patients with advanced renal cell cancers who were treated with bevacizumab and everolimus reportedly developed OM [16].

## Risk of mucositis

It is clear to anyone who takes care of cancer patients, that despite similarities in diagnosis and treatment, they are not at equal risk of developing mucositis or other toxicities. For example, we know that about 10% of patients with newly diagnosed disease have a greater than 50% chance of developing mucositis [7]. Among this group are patients who receive radiation therapy with or without chemotherapy for the treatment of cancers of the head and neck and patients treated with aggressive forms of chemotherapy, especially with total body irradiation, as conditioning regimens prior to stem cell transplant. Interestingly, even among these two groups, there are a significant number of patients who will have little or no oral mucosal injury.

Conversely, about 40% of new cancer patients will never be at risk of developing any form of clinically significant mucositis [7]. These patients are treated with surgery only, with nonstomatotoxic agents at low doses, or with focal, nonoral radiation therapy.

The largest group of patients will fall in an intermediate category in which the risk of mucositis is somewhere between 20% and 49%. Cancer diagnoses in this group are those of the most common types: breast, colorectal and lung cancer. Cycled chemotherapy is the norm in this cohort and, importantly, if a patient develops mucositis in one cycle of treatment, the risk of a repeat is over 70% in subsequent cycles [7].

## Risk determinants

What accounts for such variation? Historically, mucositis risk has been attributed to factors that are associated with treatment and those attributable to the patient. More recently, recognition that the tumor itself may play a role in mucositis risk has been reported (Figure 3.2) [17].

## Treatment-related factors

Treatment-related variables include those associated with the type of therapy, dose, and route of administration. To a large extent, treatment type and dose can be overwhelming risk factors. Thus for a patient with a tongue cancer who is receiving chemoradiation, the likelihood of mucositis is close to 100% [7]. On the other hand, a patient with a hypopharyngeal cancer, also receiving chemoradiation may see the risk drop to 50% because the tissues of the oral cavity are not primarily included in the radiation field [7]. Patients receiving conditioning regimens in preparation for HSCT have been considered to be at high risk of mucositis. As noted above, this was true of many regimens, especially those that included total body irradiation and/or high doses of stomatotoxic drugs.

## Patient-related factors

Patient-related risk factors are more complex. Among those mentioned are age, body mass, gender, pre-existing medical conditions and genetics

**Risk determinants for mucositis**

**Treatment-related**
- Type of radiation
- Site of radiation
- Radiation or chemotherapy dose and schedule
- Drug selection
- Use of adjuvant agents

**Patient-related**
- Older age
- Body mass
- Female gender
- Genes
- Oral environment

**Tumor type**

Figure 3.2 Risk determinants for mucositis.

[7,18]. For the most part these are poorly defined, although data suggests that being female confers increased toxicity risk for 5-FU [11] and methotrexate [19].

## The role of pre-existing conditions

Pre-existing conditions may impact mucositis risk. For example, in a study of patients receiving induction therapy for leukemia, patients who had psoriasis, a condition in which there is excess epithelial proliferation, were at less risk of mucositis than patients with Addison's disease, a disease in which patients have high levels of pro-inflammatory cytokines [7] (see Chapter 2).

## The role of genetic factors

It is becoming increasing clear that genetic factors play a dominant role in determining mucositis risk (Figure 3.3) [7]. Genes can impact mucositis risk on at least two levels. They can impact the enzymes that metabolize chemotherapy drugs. For example, a patient missing the portion of a gene that controls dihydropryrimidine dehydrogenase would be at increased toxicity risk from fluorouracil. Fortunately, enzymatic deficiencies are relatively rare. Rather, it seems more likely that differences in the expression of genes associated with OM pathogenesis are more likely to impact risk.

A number of examples can be found that illustrate this hypothesis. TNF-$\alpha$ appears to play a role in OM development, and a number of polymorphisms control individuals' TNF-$\alpha$ production [20]. The expression of TNF-$\alpha$ *1,2 has been found to increase toxicity risk, including mucositis, among patients undergoing allogeneic HSCT (Figure 3.4) [21].

Another example of mechanistic gene-based risk is provided by studies of radiation-induced dermatitis, a condition with a pathogenesis that is

**Genetic determinants of mucositis risk work at three levels**

| Treatment-related |
|---|
| Drug metabolism |
| Direct cell response to drug |
| Bystander biologic targets of drug |

Figure 3.3 Genetic determinants of mucositis risk work at three levels.

similar to mucositis. ROS play an important role during the initiation phase [22]. Consequently, differences in polymorphisms that encode for glutathione S-transferase (GST), an enzyme that provides protection from ROS, impact the extent of radiation-induced dermatitis. Low activity of the GSTP genotype was associated with a more than two-fold risk for acute skin toxicity [23]. Results in another study of showed that deletion polymorphisms in GST mu and theta resulted in a significant increase in toxicity risk, including mucositis. In fact the difference in mucositis frequency between patients with the polymorphisms and those without them was 74% vs. 55% (Figure 3.5) [24].

| Risk factors for severe toxicities in allogeneic hematopoietic stem cell transplants ||
| --- | --- |
| **Risk factor** | **Odds ratio** |
| Donor–recipient gender relationship (F→M) | 4.2 |
| Recipient's age | 2.1 |
| Aggressive conditioning regimen | 7.0 |
| Tumor necrosis factor-alpha *1,2 | 17.2 |

Figure 3.4 **Risk factors for severe toxicities in allogeneic hematopoietic stem cell transplants.** As noted in Chapter 2, tumor necrosis factor (TNF) appears to play a role in the development of mucositis and other toxicities. In Bogunia-Kubik's study, patients with the TNF-alphaα *1,2 genotype were at much higher risk of toxicities associated with conditioning regimens for hematopoietic stem cell transplants than were individuals without the genotype. Data from Bogunia-Kubik et al [21].

| Relative risk estimate for Grade 2–4 RRT polymorphisms associated with glutathione-S-transferase |||
| --- | --- | --- |
| **Polymorphism** | **Relative risk** | **Significance** |
| Absence GSTM1 | 1.59 | Not significant |
| Absence GSTT1 | 1.25 | Not significant |
| Presence both GSTM1 and GSTT1 | 1.87 | $P=0.035$ |

Figure 3.5 **Relative risk estimate for Grade 2–4 RRT polymorphisms associated with glutathione-S-transferase.** An example of how functional polymorphisms can impact the risk of oral mucositis. Reactive oxygen species (ROS) are important drivers of mucositis (Chapter 2). Hahn and her colleagues studied the impact of a deletion polymorphism that resulted in an absence of glutathione-S-transferase, the enzyme that typically neutralizes ROS. They found that the presence of either of the genes, which exhibit the deletion polymorphism resulted in an increase in the relative risk of toxicity. While these were not significant when expressed individually, when they both occurred together, significant risk increase was observed. Ulcerative mucositis was the most common toxicity noted in their study and its risk was markedly affected by the presence of the studied polymorphisms. GSTM, glutathione-S-transferase mu; GSTT, glutathione-S-transferase theta. Data from Hahn et al [24].

## Tumor-related factors

Too often we forget that the tumor itself is biologically active and might contribute to OM risk. There is significant data to suggest that both the tumor's parenchyma and stroma are sources of molecules, which influence cell behavior and impact toxicity risk [25]. For example, tumor-derived peptides and protein products could directly modify normal cell response to radiation or chemotherapy or enhance the breakdown of the local tissue environment. The role of the tumor as a risk modifier requires much additional study.

# The oral environment and mucositis

The environment in which the oral mucosa sits cannot be ignored and has an impact on the course of mucositis. The oral cavity is one of the most complex environments in the body. The oral microbial flora consist of bacteria, fungi, and viruses, all of which are impacted by the local and systemic state of the patient.

## Saliva

While the role of saliva in the development and course of OM deserves additional study, treatments aimed at stimulating salivary flow as OM treatments have largely failed [26,27].

## Bacteria

We know that the normal bacterial flora undergo changes in myelosuppressed patients [28]. Increases in gram negative organisms have been documented and, most recently, increases in organisms traditionally associated with skin (staphylococci) have been reported. While it seems quite clear that mucositis is not an infectious disease, the ability of organisms to colonize ulcerated surfaces (Figure 3.6) and secrete biologically active products means that their presence can result in secondary local effects.

## Fungi and viruses

Fungi and viruses that are typically associated with mucosal injury have been aggressively studied for their potential involvement in the development of mucositis. In particular, *Candida albicans* infection, common in radiated patients with xerostomia, seems to be a concurrent, but not etiologic component of mucositis in this patient population. Antifungals as mucositis interventions have not been effective [29], a finding that is not surprising given the large number of patients who develop mucositis even when they receive routine antifungal prophylaxis.

Speculation that the herpes simplex virus (HSV) might be a cause of mucositis first emerged in the 1980s [30]. However, since that time a range of data based on cultures, antibody status and efficacy of antiviral therapy have led to the conclusion that HSV is not associated with the development of mucositis [31]. Nonetheless, since it is possible for patients to have concurrent fungal or viral infections, their presence should not be arbitrarily dismissed, especially in myelosuppressed individuals (see Chapter 9).

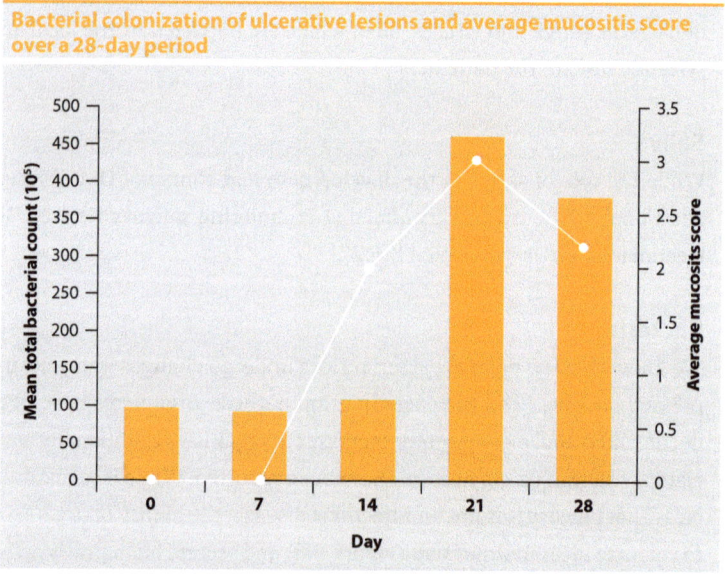

**Bacterial colonization of ulcerative lesions and average mucositis score over a 28-day period**

Figure 3.6 **Bacterial colonization of ulcerative lesions and average mucositis score over a 28-day period.** The relationship between mucositis severity (graph) and bacterial colonization (bars). The relationship between quantitative increases in bacteria and the course of mucositis was studied in a hamster model in which an acute dose of radiation was given on day 0. Bacterial sampling and clinical mucositis scoring was performed at weekly intervals. Mucositis development (a score of three indicates ulcerative OM) preceded increases in bacterial numbers suggesting that, at least quantitatively, bacteria do not drive the development of mucosal ulceration. Bacterial colonization of ulcerative lesions is suggested by the synchronous peak of mean bacterial count and mucositis score on day 21. Reproduced with permission from Sonis [7].

# References

1 Sun CC, Bodurka DC, Weaver CB, et al. Rankings and symptom assessments of side effects from chemotherapy: insights from experienced patients with ovarian cancer. *Support Care Cancer*. 2005; 13: 219-227.

2 Elting LS, Cooksley CD, Chambers MS, Garden AS. Risk, outcomes, and costs of radiation-induced oral mucositis among patients with head-and-neck malignancies. *Int J Radiat Oncol Biol Phys*. 2007;68:1110-1120.

3 Treister N, Sonis S. Oral mucositis. In: Ettinger DS, ed. *Cancer and Drug Discovery Development: Supportive Care in Cancer Therapy*. Totowa, NJ: Humana Press. 2008;193-211.

4 Blijlevens N, Schwenkglenks M, Bacon P, et al. Prospective oral mucositis audit: oral mucositis in patients receiving high-dose melphalan or BEAM conditioning chemotherapy - European Blood and Marrow Transplantation Mucositis Advisory Group. *J Clin Oncol*. 2008;261519-1525.

5 Spielberger R, Stiff P, Bensinger W, et al. Palifermin for oral mucositis after intensive therapy for hematologic cancers. *N Engl J Med*. 2004;351:2590-2598.

6 Sonis ST. A biological approach to mucositis. *J Support Oncol*. 2004;2:21-32.

7 Sonis ST. Mucositis: The impact, biology and therapeutic opportunities of oral mucositis. *Oral Oncol*. 2009;45:1015-1020.

8 Chan S, Romieu G, Huober J, et al. Phase III study of gemcitabine plus docetaxel compared with capecitabine plus docetaxel for anthracycline-pretreated patients with metastatic breast cancer. *J Clin Oncol*. 2009;27:1753-1760.

9 Keefe DM, Schubert MM, Elting LS, et al. Updated clinical practice guidelines for the prevention and treatment of mucositis. *Cancer*. 2007;109:820-831.

10 Grunberg S, Hesketh P, Randolph-Jackson P, et al. Risk, quality of life impact of mucosal injury among colorectal cancer patients receiving FOLFOX chemotherapy. *Support Care Cancer*. 2007;15:704.

11 Sloan JA, Loprinzi CL, Novotny PJ, et al. Sex differences in fluorouracil-induced stomatitis. *J Clin Oncol*. 2000;18:412-420.

12 Faderl S, Garcia-Manero G, Estrov Z, et al. Oral clofarabine in the treatment of patients with higher risk myelodysplastic syndrome. *J Clin Oncol*. 2010;28:2755-2760.

13 Malik SM, Liu K, Qiang X, et al. Folotyn (pralatrexate injection) for the treatment of patients with relapsed or refractory peripheral T-cell lymphoma: US Food and Drug Administration drug approval summary. *Clin Cancer Res*. 2010;16:4921-4927.

14 Krzakowski M, Ramlau R, Jassem J, et al. Phase III trial comparing vinflunine with docetaxel in second-line advanced non-small-cell lung cancer previously treated with platinumcontaining chemotherapy. *J Clin Oncol*. 2010;28:2167-2173.

15 O'Donnell A, Faivre S, Burris HA, et al. Phase I pharmacokinetic and pharmacodynamic study of the oral mammalian target of rapamycin inhibitor everolimus in patients with advanced solid tumors. *J Clin Oncol*. 2008;26:1588-1595.

16 Hainsworth JD, Spigel DR, Burris HA, et al. Phase II trial of bevacizumab and everolimus in patients with advanced renal cell cancer. *J Clin Oncol*. 2010;28:2131-2136.

17 Sonis ST. Keynote address MASCC/ISOO International Symposium 2008, Houston Texas, USA.

18 Barasch A, Peterson DE. Risk factors for ulcerative oral mucositis in cancer patients: unanswered questions. *Oral Oncol*. 2003;39:91-100.

19 Igawa M, Kadena H, Ueda M, Usui T. Association between patient characteristics and treatment history, and toxicity associated with methotrexate, vinblastine, adriamycin and cisplatin (M-VAC) for advanced urothelial cancer. *Br J Urol*. 1994;73:263-267.

20 Logan RM, Stringer AM, Bowen JM, et al. Serum levels of NFkappaB and pro-inflammatory cytokines following administration of mucotoxic drugs. *Cancer Biol Ther*. 2008;7:1139-1145.

21 Bogunia-Kubik K, Polak M, Lange A. TNF polymorphisms are associated with toxic but not with aGVHD complications in the recipients of allogeneic sibling haematopoietic stem cell transplantation. *Bone Marrow Transplan*. 2003;32:617-622.

22 Sonis ST. Oral mucositis in cancer therapy. *J Support Oncol*. 2004;2(suppl 3):3-8.

23  Ambrosone CB, Tian C, Ahn J, et al. Genetic predictors of acute toxicities related to radiation therapy following lumpectomy for breast cancer: a case-series study. *Breast Cancer Res.* 2006;8:R40.

24  Hahn T, Zhelnova E, Sucheston L, et al. A deletion polymorphism in glutathione-S-transferase mu (GSTM1) and/or theta (GSTT1) is associated with an increased risk of toxicity after autologous blood and marrow transplantation. *Biol Blood Marrow Transplant.* 2010;16:801-808.

25  Meirovitz A, Kuten M, Billan S, et al. Cytokine levels, severity of acute mucositis and the need of PEG tube installation during chemo-radiation for head and neck cancer – a prospective pilot study. *Radiation Oncol.* 2010;5:16.

26  Scarantino C, LeVeque F, Swann RS, et al. Effect of pilocarpine during radiation therapy: results of RTOG97-09, a phase III, randomized study in head and neck cancer patients. *J Support Oncol.* 2006;4:252-258.

27  Lockhart PB, Brennan MT, Kent ML, et al. Randomized controlled trial of pilocarpine hydrochloride for the moderation of oral mucositis during autologous blood stem cell transplantation. *Bone Marrow Transplant.* 2005;35:713-720.

28  Donnelly JP, Bellm LA, Epstein JB, et al. Antimicrobial therapy to prevent or treat oral mucositis. *Lancet Infect Dis.* 2003;3:405-412.

29  El-Sayed S, Nabid A, Shelley W, et al. Prophylaxis of radiation-associated mucositis in conventionally treated patients with head and neck cancer: a double-blind, phase III, randomized, controlled trial evaluating the clinical efficacy of an antimicrobial lozenge using a validated mucositis scoring system. *J Clin Oncol.* 2002;20:3956-3963.

30  Peterson DE. Oral complications associated with hematologic neoplasms and their treatment. In: Peterson DE, Elias EG, Sonis ST, eds. *Head and Neck Management of the Cancer Patient.* Boston, MA: Martinus Nijhoff; 1986:351-360.

31  Woo SB, Sonis ST, Sonis AL. The role of herpes simplex virus in the development of oral mucositis in bone marrow transplant recipients. *Cancer.* 1990;66:2375-2379.

Development of this book was supported by funding from Helsinn

# Chapter 4

# Health and economic consequences of mucositis

Pain is the most universal symptom associated with mucositis. Numerous studies have documented its relationship to clinically assessed mucositis severity, although the variability of scoring criteria (see Chapter 6) has resulted in some scales having more concordance with patient-reported pain than others. Nonetheless, data supporting a strong association between the course of clinically reported mucositis and the level of patient-reported pain are compelling [1]. For example, Figure 4.1 shows the correlation between mucositis severity as graded by National Cancer Institute Common Toxicity Criteria (NCI-CTC), patient-reported mouth pain, and dysphagia as reported by Cella and colleagues in a study of 323 patients receiving stomatotoxic chemotherapy (Figure 4.1) [2].

While the impact of OM often focuses on the causality of the severe mouth pain that it inflicts, it is also associated with a range of undesirable outcomes that affect patients' quality of life, their use of health resources, the overall cost of their cancer therapy and, ultimately, their ability to tolerate treatment.

## Patient quality of life

It has become increasingly clear that mucositis adversely affects patients' quality of life. Studies in which mucositis severity and quality of life outcomes are simultaneously tracked consistently demonstrate a correlation between the two. In a recent prospective study of 126 patients treated for cancers of the head and neck, Elting and

S. T. Sonis, *Oral Mucositis*,
DOI: 10.1007/978-1-907673-46-7_4, © Springer Healthcare 2012

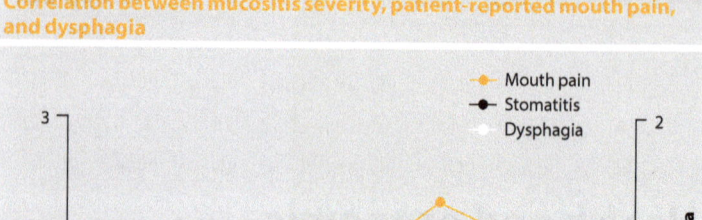

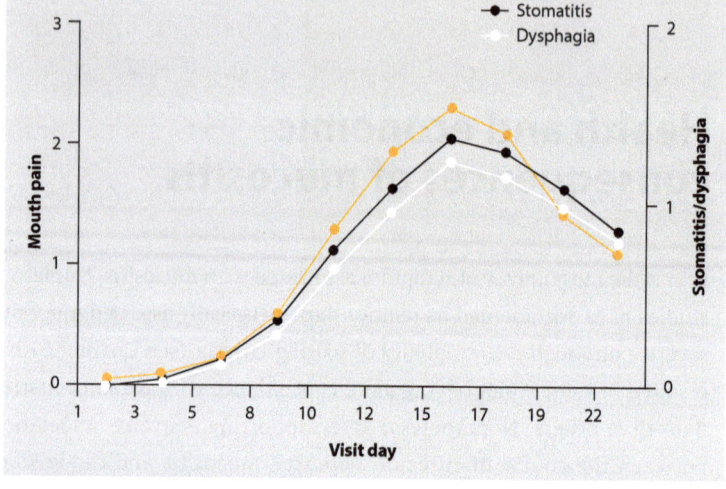

**Figure 4.1 Correlation between mucositis severity, patient-reported mouth pain, and dysphagia.** Mucositis is associated with mouth pain, and dysphagia. In the 323 patients who were being treated for hematological malignancies, Cella and colleagues found that symptoms tracked closely to the clinical findings associated with mucositis. Reproduced with permission from Cella et al [2].

colleagues demonstrated that even mild mucositis was associated with reduced quality of life measurements such as patients' senses of physical, emotional, social, and functional well-being [3].

## Increased use of health resources

Studies of patients being treated for cancers of the head and neck have provided data that demonstrate the relationship of mucositis to undesirable outcomes and an increased use of health resources.

A study of more than 400 patients being treated with chemoradiation for cancers of the head and neck compared differences in six resource use outcomes (Figure 4.2) [4]. Increasing severity of mucositis was associated with significant increases in the inability of patients to comply with planned treatment, use of parenteral or enteral feeding, placement and use of indwelling intravenous access, and hospitalization.

**Severity of mucositis in patients with head and neck cancer**

| | Severity of oral mucositis | | | | | |
|---|---|---|---|---|---|---|
| **Outcome** | **None (n=75)** | **Mild (n=83)** | **Moderate (n=152)** | **Severe (n=124)** | **P** | **Odds ratio** |
| Radiotherapy | 12 (16%) | 19 (24%) | 48 (32%) | 73 (59%) | <0.001 | 3.8 |
| + Chemotherapy | 5 (16%) | 5 (21%) | 17 (27%) | 37 (56%) | <0.001 | 3.4 |
| Chemotherapy dose reduction | 1 (3%) | 1 (3%) | 8 (13%) | 11 (16%) | 0.001 | 6.1 |
| Feeding tube/ total parenteral nutrition (other than prophylaxis) | 8 (11 %) | 6 (7%) | 22 (14%) | 25 (19%) | 0.009 | 1.8 |
| Indwelling intravenous catheter | 15 (20%) | 14 (17%) | 40 (26%) | 45 (35%) | 0.013 | 1.9 |
| Hospitalization | 8 (11%) | 17 (20%) | 24 (16%) | 42 (33%) | <0.001 | 3.5 |

**Figure 4.2 Severity of mucositis in patients with head and neck cancer.** As the severity of mucositis increases, so does the frequency of treatment modifications and resource use. For example, in a retrospective study of 400 patients being treated for cancers of the head and neck in a range of practice settings, Vera-Llonch and collaborators found that outcomes such as unplanned breaks or delays in treatment, feeding tube use, and hospitalizations were highly impacted by the severity of the patient's mucositis. Data from Vera-Llonch et al [4].

## Overall cost of cancer therapy

Healthcare costs are increasingly being scrutinized. To assess the financial impact of mucositis, resource use was compared between patients with or without mucositis who were being treated for cancers of the lung or head and neck. Unlike the data presented above, these data simply dichotomized outcomes between patients who had mucositis and those who did not. The results are dramatic with the incremental costs of mucositis being more than $17,000 (US) (Figure 4.3) [5].

Not unexpectedly, the biggest driver of increased cost was attributable to the cost of hospitalization. This is especially dramatic in patient populations that are typically treated in an ambulatory setting, such as those receiving radiation therapy or conventional cycled chemotherapy. Once a patient passes the hospital admission threshold (in the mucositis population usually for hydration, pain or infection management), additional costs accrue rapidly and are primarily associated with diagnostic procedures. Figure 4.3 only reflects treatment costs that are directly related to the management of mucositis, not concordant conditions. Additional

**Impact of oral mucositis on treatment costs in head and neck cancer and nonsmall-cell lung cancer**

| Sources of direct medical cost | Without oral mucositis (US $) (n= 54) | With oral mucositis (US $) (n=85) | Incremental cost for patients with mucositis (US $) (n=139) |
|---|---|---|---|
| Inpatient hospitalization | 7000 | 19,600 | 12,600 |
| Tests and procedures | 1094 | 3419 | 2325 |
| Imaging procedures | 5900 | 7019 | 1119 |
| Clinical visits | 1080 | 1500 | 420 |
| Mucositis-related medication | 84 | 195 | 110 |
| Diagnostic tests | 494 | 595 | 101 |
| **Total** | **20,798** | **39,313** | **18,515** |

**Figure 4.3 Impact of oral mucositis on treatment costs in head and neck cancer and nonsmall-cell lung cancer.** Median direct costs of treatment. We live in an era of healthcare cost containment. As shown by Nonzee and coworkers, among patients being treated for cancers of the lung and head and neck, mucositis added significant incremental costs to care. The most important events which contributed to this difference were hospitalizations and the tests and diagnostic procedures that followed. This retrospective study evaluated patients treated in a VA hospital, a county hospital, and a comprehensive cancer center. Data from Nonzee et al [5].

mucositis-associated costs in patients being treated as outpatients for their cancers are attributable to their increased need for unplanned office visits or visits to the emergency room.

In contrast, patients receiving HSCTs are typically hospitalized. Despite this though, mucositis is also a cause of increased resource use and cost. This result is largely a function of the fact that many of the conditioning regimens delivered prior to HSCT simultaneously result in mucositis and myelosuppression. As a consequence, the risk of secondary infection of ulcerated mucosa or systemic infection of oral origin is increased and with it, the cost of management. A comparison of the difference in the number of days of health outcome use between HSCT patients with or without mucositis is illustrative (Figure 4.4) [6]. From the standpoint of cost, the most important factor is the observation that patients with ulcerative mucositis have longer hospital stays than patients who do not develop the condition. It has been estimated that the incremental cost for ulcerative mucositis in this patient cohort exceeded $40,000 (US) [6].

**Impact of mucositis on bad health and economic outcomes in hematopoietic stem cell transplant patients**

| Health outcome | Increase in days for patients with oral mucositis compared with those without oral mucositis | P |
|---|---|---|
| Days of injectable narcotics | 4.80 | <0.01 |
| Days of total parenteral nutrition | 5.34 | <0.01 |
| Febrile days | 1.59 | <0.02 |
| Days with significant infection | 2.55 | <0.05 |
| Hospital days (autologous HSCT) | 11.02 | <0.01 |
| Hospital days (allogeneic HSCT) | 6.92 | <0.02 |

**Figure 4.4 Impact of mucositis on bad health and economic outcomes in hematopoietic stem cell transplant patients.** Unlike patients being treated for head and neck cancer, patients who receive HSCT are hospitalized from the start. Many of the conditioning regimens used in preparation of HSCT are stomatotoxic and patients who develop mucositis require more care and treatment than those that do not. The data above show the differences in the numbers of days of resource use between patients who developed mucositis and those who did not. As a consequence, the impact of mucositis on cost of care was estimated to exceed $40,000 (US). The data are based on an evaluation of 92 subjects from 8 cancer centers who were participants in a study, which validated the Oral Mucositis Assessment Scale. HSCT, hematopoietic stem cell transplant. Data from Sonis et al [6].

The overall health and economic costs for OM in patients receiving cycled chemotherapy for the most common malignancies has not been well studied. Furthermore, the impact of newer targeted therapies on altering mucositis-driven resource use has yet to be explored.

# References

1   Wong PC, Dodd MJ, Miaskowski C, et al. Mucositis pain induced by radiation therapy: prevalence, severity, and use of self-care behaviors. *J Pain Symptom Manage*. 2006;32:27-37.
2   Cella D, Pulliam J, Fuchs H, et al. Evaluation of pain associated with oral mucositis during the acute period after administration of high-dose chemotherapy. *Cancer*. 2003;98:406-412.
3   Elting LS, Keefe DM, Sonis ST, et al. Patient-reported measurements of oral mucositis in head and neck cancer patients treated with radiotherapy with or without chemotherapy: demonstration of increased frequency, severity, resistance to palliation, and impact on quality of life. *Cancer*. 2008;113:2704-2713.
4   Vera-Llonch M, Oster G, Hagiwara M, Sonis S. Oral mucositis in patients undergoing radiation treatment for head and neck carcinoma. *Cancer*. 2006;106:329-336.
5   Nonzee NJ, Dandade NA, Patel U, et al. Evaluating the supportive care costs of severe radiochemotherapy-induced mucositis and pharyngitis: results from a Northwestern University Costs of Cancer Program pilot study with head and neck and nonsmall cell lung cancer patients who received care at a county hospital, a Veterans Administration hospital, or a comprehensive cancer care center. *Cancer*. 2008;113:1446-1452.
6   Sonis ST, Oster G, Fuchs H, et al. Oral mucositis and the clinical and economic outcomes of hematopoietic stem-cell transplantation. *J Clin Oncol*. 2001;19:2201-2205.

Development of this book was supported by funding from Helsinn

# Chapter 5

# The elements of examination of the oral cavity

## Introduction and sequence

The clinical examination of the oral cavity is straightforward and easily accomplished with minimum tissue manipulation or discomfort to patients. As with any physical examination, a standardized sequence and good lighting are important to assure accuracy. The procedure should take no more than two minutes to complete.

OM can occur on any aspect of the movable oral mucosa – there are no sentinel sites, although lesions are most prevalent on the buccal mucosa (Figure 5.1) and lateral and ventral tongue surfaces (Figure 5.2).

Mucositis does not occur on the more heavily keratinized areas of the mouth such as the hard palate, dorsal tongue, or gingiva. Nonetheless, the examination should include these sites as they are common areas for both fungal (candidiasis) and viral infections (see Chapter 8).

An examination sequence that has had good success in assessing OM is the following:

1. Mandibular labial mucosa
2. Maxillary labial mucosa
3. Right buccal mucosa
4. Left buccal mucosa
5. Right lateral and ventral tongue
6. Left lateral and ventral tongue
7. Floor of the mouth
8. Soft palate
9. Hard palate

S. T. Sonis, *Oral Mucositis*,
DOI: 10.1007/978-1-907673-46-7_5, © Springer Healthcare 2012

### Oral mucositis on the movable buccal mucosa

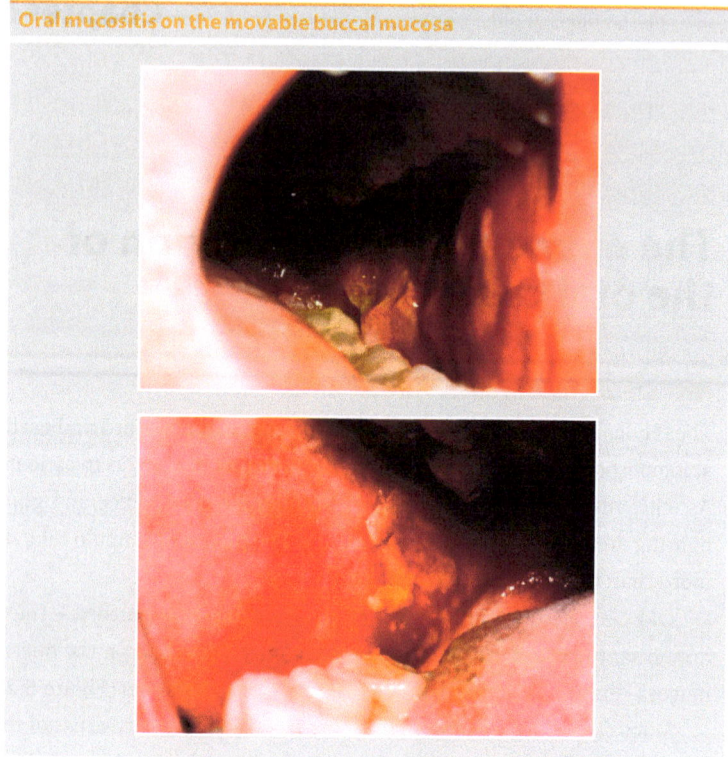

**Figure 5.1 Oral mucositis on the movable buccal mucosa.** Good lighting enhances the examiner's ability to assess the mouth. These two images are of the same patient, but with different lighting.

### Prevalence of ulcers by site

| Site | % Ulceration |
| --- | --- |
| Upper lip | 4.7 |
| Lower lip | 7.0 |
| Right cheek | 16.6 |
| Left cheek | 16.9 |
| Right ventral and lateral tongue | 19.1 |
| Left ventral and lateral tongue | 18.7 |
| Floor of mouth | 10.0 |
| Soft palate | 6.9 |

**Figure 5.2 Prevalence of ulcers by site.** There is no sentinel site for mucositis. It may occur on aspects of the movable oral mucosa. The most common sites include the tongue and buccal mucosa, but the lesions of the soft palate are among the most painful.

## Armamentarium

Good lighting is essential to assuring an accurate examination. While handheld penlights or flashlights are traditional and will work, they eliminate the opportunity for the examiner to use two hands. This is a drawback particularly when tissue retraction is essential for site visualization as is required for examination of the buccal or labial mucosa or tongue.

An inexpensive alternative is to use a headlamp such as those used by campers (Figure 5.3). These lights are battery operated, totally portable, easily fit into a lab coat pocket, and lightweight. A word of caution however – when using a light, shine it onto your palm to localize the beam. Otherwise you risk shining the light into your patient's eyes.

Aside from a light, you will need examination gloves, a wooden tongue depressor, and a gauze sponge (Figure 5.3).

**Armamentarium for clinical examination of the buccal cavity**

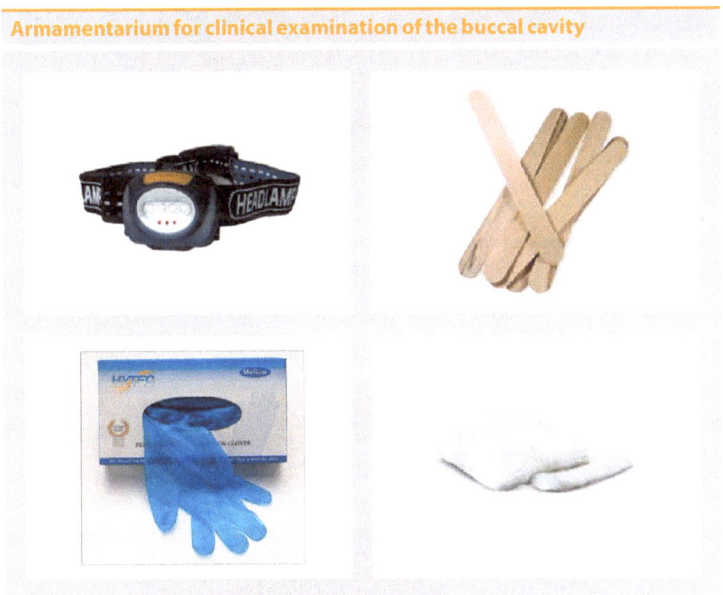

**Figure 5.3 Armamentarium for clinical examination of the buccal cavity.** An experienced examiner should be able to perform a thorough examination of all aspects of the oral mucosa and oropharynx in under two minutes. A headlight not only provides good illumination, it frees up the hands to manipulate tissue and enhance visualization. Headlights can be purchased inexpensively through any camping supplier. Square gauze sponges are helpful in holding the tongue to examine the lateral borders and in drying saliva.

## Examination of the oral cavity

Begin by grasping the upper lip and gently lifting to expose the gingiva, alveolar mucosa and labial mucosa (Figure 5.4). Repeat the process for the lower lip (Figure 5.5). Using the tongue blade, gently retract the right cheek to expose the buccal mucosa. Your ability to visualize the whole surface all the way back to the mandible will be enhanced by having the patient close slightly as this will loosen the facial muscles. The parotid duct should be visualized on the buccal mucosa opposite

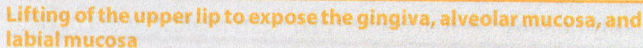

Lifting of the upper lip to expose the gingiva, alveolar mucosa, and labial mucosa

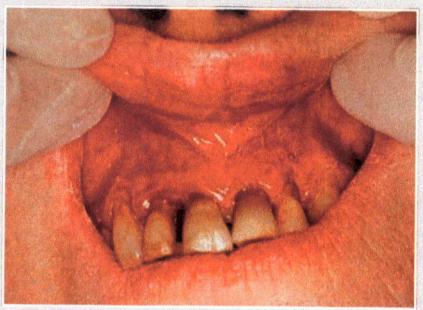

**Figure 5.4 Lifting of the upper lip to expose the gingiva, alveolar mucosa, and labial mucosa.** As is the case with components of the physical examination of a patient, sticking to a regular sequence minimizes the risk of missing or forgetting a site.

Lifting of the lower lip to expose the gingiva, alveolar mucosa, and labial mucosa

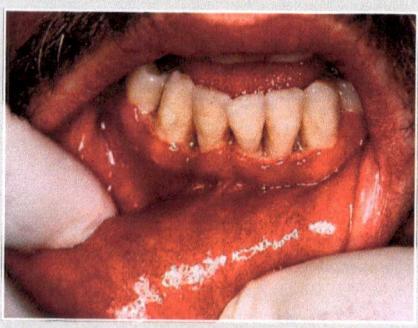

**Figure 5.5 Lifting of the lower lip to expose the gingiva, alveolar mucosa, and labial mucosa.**

the maxillary second molar (Figure 5.6). Repeat the process for the left buccal mucosa (Figure 5.7).

Using a cotton gauze sponge, grasp the tongue, gently pull it out of the patient's mouth and roll it first to the left to visualize the right lateral and ventral surfaces, and then to the right to view the left lateral and ventral surfaces (Figure 5.8).

To view the floor of the mouth, simply ask the patient to touch the tongue to the roof of the mouth. The submandibular ducts should be easily visualized (Figure 5.9).

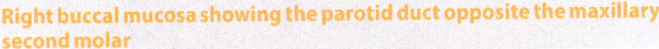

**Right buccal mucosa showing the parotid duct opposite the maxillary second molar**

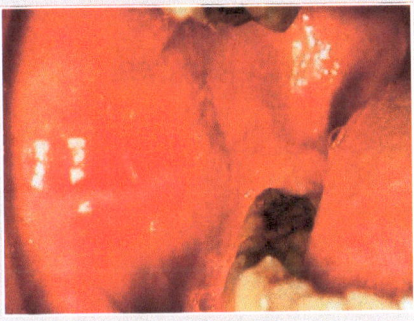

**Figure 5.6 Right buccal mucosa showing the parotid duct opposite the maxillary second molar.**

**Left buccal mucosa**

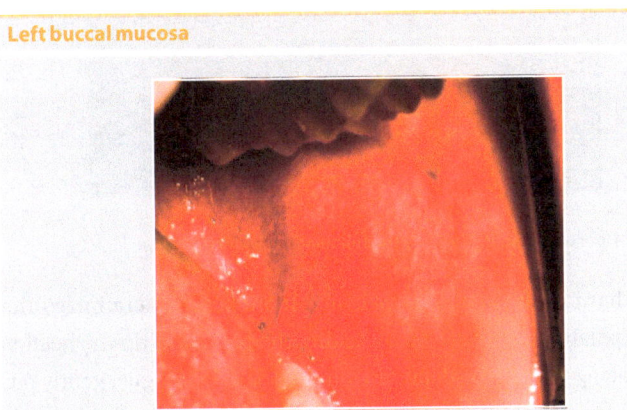

**Figure 5.7 Left buccal mucosa.**

## Lateral and ventral surface of the tongue

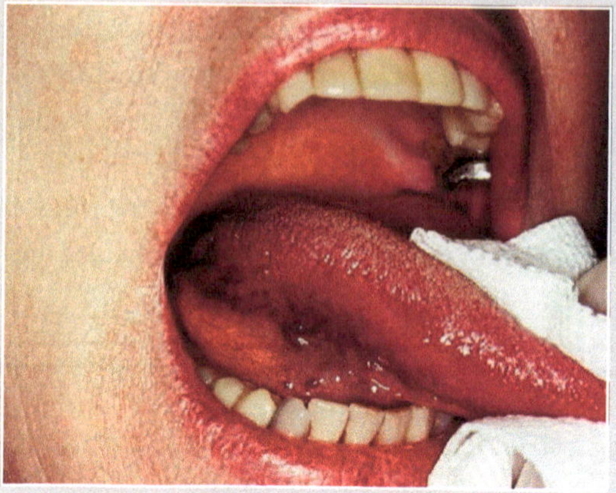

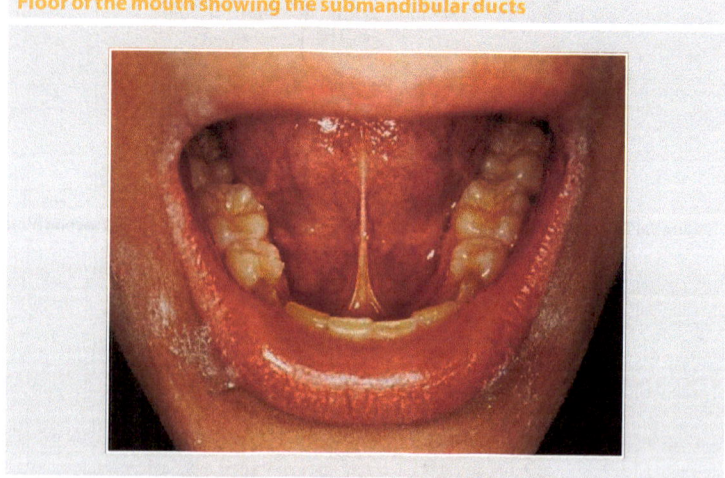

Figure 5.8 Lateral and ventral surface of the tongue.

## Floor of the mouth showing the submandibular ducts

Figure 5.9 Floor of the mouth showing the submandibular ducts.

The hard palate is nonmovable and more heavily keratinized than the soft palate. It can be seen by asking the patient to tip the head up. After placing the tongue depressor on the posterior tongue, gently push forward and ask the patient to constrict the palatal muscles by saying ahhh to view the soft palate and uvula (Figure 5.10).

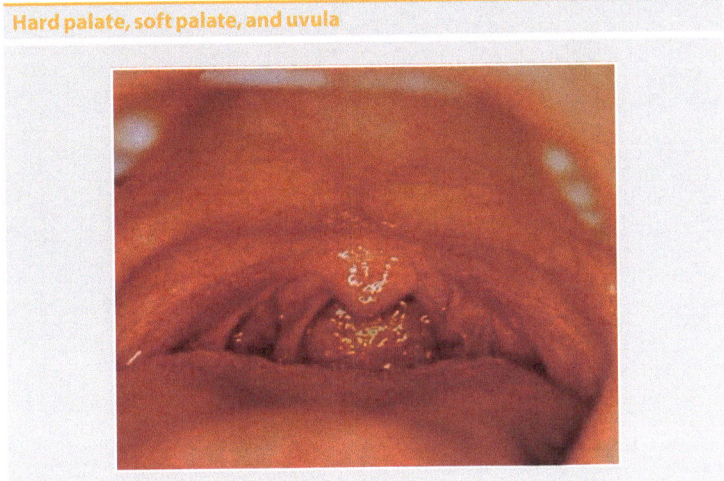

**Figure 5.10 Hard palate, soft palate, and uvula.**

## Examination of children

Like adults, children get mucositis. While the same anatomic sites need to be evaluated, the examination technique can be modified slightly to account for smaller mouths. A pediatric throat stick can be used or ignored in favor of a gloved finger to gently retract the tongue. Most importantly, the examiner should communicate continuously with the child to explain what she or he is doing and provide reassurance and praise.

Development of this book was supported by funding from Helsinn

# Chapter 6

# A comparison and assessment of scoring scales for mucositis

The presence and severity of OM may be determined by clinician-based scoring or by patient-reported endpoints. This chapter will focus on clinician-based scoring scales. Patient-reported outcomes are described in Chapter 7.

There are three major reasons to assess mucositis severity:

1. To determine the stomatotoxicity of a particular cancer-treatment regimen
2. To help in the management of the patient
3. As a research tool to evaluate the efficacy of a potential mucositis intervention

## Toxicity description and assessment

Scoring scales to describe toxicity are among the most common and include those that use National Cancer Institute Common Toxicity Criteria (NCI-CTC), Radiation Therapy Oncology Group (RTOG), and World Health Organization (WHO) criteria to assess mucositis severity (Figure 6.1) [1]. These scores are then used to describe the overall toxicity of a particular chemotherapy regimen or radiation schedule. To a large degree, these scales are focused on clinician examination of the oral mucosa and the assignment of a score based on observed clinical changes such as erythema and ulceration. They may also have a component that is based on patient function or use of analgesics.

S. T. Sonis, *Oral Mucositis*,
DOI: 10.1007/978-1-907673-46-7_6, © Springer Healthcare 2012

**Toxicity grading of oral mucositis according to different grading schemes**

| Scale | Side effect(s) | Grade 0 (none) | Grade 1 (mild) | Grade 2 (moderate) | Grade 3 (severe) | Grade 4 (life-threatening) | Grade 5 (death) |
|---|---|---|---|---|---|---|---|
| WHO | Oral mucositis (stomatitis) | None | Oral soreness, erythema | Oral erythema, ulcers, solid diet tolerated | Oral ulcers, liquid diet only | Oral alimentation impossible | – |
| NCI-CTC | Chemotherapy-induced stomatitis/pharyngitis (oral/pharyngeal mucositis) | None | Painless ulcers, erythema, or mild soreness in the absence of lesions | Painful erythema, edema, or ulcers but eating or swallowing possible | Painful erythema, edema, or ulcers requiring intravenous hydration | Severe ulceration or requiring parenteral or enteral nutritional support or prophylactic intubation | Death related to toxicity |
| NCI-CTC | Associated with HSCT (stomatitis/pharyngitis, oral/pharyngeal mucositis) | None | Painless ulcers, erythema, or mild soreness in the absence of lesions | Painful erythema, edema, or ulcers but swallowing possible | Painful erythema, edema, or ulcers preventing swallowing or requiring hydration or parenteral (or enteral) nutritional support | Severe ulceration requiring prophylactic intubation or resulting in documented aspiration pneumonia | Death related to toxicity |
| NCI-CTC | Mucositis due to radiation | None | Erythema of the mucosa | Patchy, pseudomembranous reaction (patches generally <1.5 cm in greatest dimension and noncontiguous) | Pseudo-membranous reaction (contiguous patches generally >1.5 cm in greatest dimension) | Ulceration and occasional bleeding not induced by minor trauma or abrasion | Death related to toxicity |
| RTOG | Acute oral mucous membrane toxicity caused by radiation | No change over baseline | Injection, may experience mild pain not requiring analgesic | Patchy mucositis that may produce inflammatory serosanguinitis discharge; may experience moderate pain requiring analgesia | Confluent, fibrinous mucositis, may include severe pain requiring narcotic | Ulceration, hemorrhage, or necrosis | – |

**Figure 6.1 Toxicity grading of oral mucositis according to different grading schemes.** HSCT, hematopoietic stem cell transplant; NCI-CTC, National Cancer Institute Common Toxicity Criteria; RTOG, Radiation Therapy Oncology Group; WHO, World Health Organization. Reproduced with permission from Sonis et al [1].

## Patient management scales

Patient management scales tend to be based on a holistic and composite evaluation of the patient's oral health, of which only one element is mucosal damage. They have been primarily developed by nurses for the daily care of their patients (Figure 6.2).

These instruments often include assessments of patient speech, salivary function and quality, gingival health, swallowing, lips, and oral hygiene. While of great value in formulating treatment plans that focus on overall oral cavity health, the evaluation of the oral mucosa is not the primary target of these scales. Examples are the Oral Assessment Guide (OAG) [2], the Western Consortium for Cancer Nursing Research (WCCNR) [3], the MacDibbs scales [4] and the Nijmegen Nursing Mucositis Scoring System (NNMSS) (Figure 6.3) [5].

## Research directed scales

Over the years, scales have been developed to be used primarily in mucositis research studies (Figure 6.4). These tend to provide highly quantitative outputs that are based on a series of strictly defined parameters. The two most commonly cited scales of this type are the Oral Mucositis Index (OMI) and the Oral Mucositis Assessment Scale (OMAS) [6] (Figure 6.5). The endpoints for both scales are dependent of clinician assessment. While the OMAS tends to be very focused on mucosal changes, the OMI has broader criteria.

---

**Patient management tools**

- Examples: Oral Assessment Guide, Western Consortium for Cancer Nursing Research
- Holistic
- Include several variables that are irrelevant to mucositis, so may over-report
- Incorporated in many nursing mouthcare standard operating procedures
- Valuable for daily assessment of oral status, but excessive number of variables dilutes value for clinical trials

**Figure 6.2 Patient management tools.** Patient management tools are typically used for assessment of the entire mouth in an effort to assure practices that lead to overall oral health. The clinical features of mucositis are typically only a single element of the scale. Thus nonmucositis components such as gingival changes, salivary consistency, speech characteristics and oral hygiene may all contribute to an aggregate score. For interventional studies, these scales are of value in assessing overall mouth symptoms and changes, but because of their global nature may not be the best choice for studying the efficacy of mucositis interventions.

## Nijmegen nursing mucositis scoring system

| | Characteristic | 0 point | 1 point | 2 points | 3 points |
|---|---|---|---|---|---|
| **Objective characteristics of oral mucositis based on oral inspection by nurse** | Erythema | Pink and moist | Mild/ moderate | Severe | |
| | Edema | Absent | Mild | Moderate | Severe |
| | | | Print of teeth in tongue edge | Print of teeth in tongue edge | Swollen tongue |
| | | | Gingival swollen and red | Gingival swollen and white | Gingival swollen and shining white |
| | | | | | Elapse ulceration |
| | Lesions | Absent | 1 to 4 | >4 | |
| **Subjective characteristics of oral mucositis based on patient-provided information** | Pain | None | VAS score <3 | VAS score 4, 5, 6 | VAS score >6 |
| | Dryness of mouth | Normal | Mild | Moderate | Severe |
| | Saliva viscosity | Normal | Slimy | Thick | |

**Figure 6.3 Nijmegen nursing mucositis scoring system.** The Nijmegen nursing mucositis scoring system is one of the most directed (from the standpoint of mucositis) of the many management scales available. Nonetheless, the scale contains scoring targets such as mouth dryness, gingival condition, and salivary viscosity, that are supplemental to the primary clinical changes of mucositis. The scale relies on clinical grading by a nurse and completion of questions regarding symptom severity by patients. A visual analog scale (VAS) for pain is also completed by the patient. The VAS consists of a 10 cm line with the extremes of the condition being evaluated at either end (eg. no pain and worst possible pain). The patient is asked to place a mark on the line which indicates how their mouth feels. Reproduced with permission from Potting et al [5].

## Mucositis research instruments

- No uniformity in end points
- Wide range of complexity
- Include several variables which are irrelevant to mucositis, so may over-report
- Major value in phase 2 trials and outcome analyses, but of limited value in phase 3 trials

**Figure 6.4 Mucositis research instruments.** Mucositis research scales were developed in an attempt to provide quantitative, highly objective endpoints for mucositis assessment. They vary widely in complexity from a 34-item Oral Mucositis Index [7], to a 16-item scale [8] to an Oral Mucositis Assessment Scale that evaluates ulceration and erythema [6]. These scales all share quantitative outcomes to which statistical analyses can be easily applied. However, the interpretation of data by clinicians is often difficult. Consequently, they are best used in focused applications.

| Oral Mucositis Assessment Scale | |
| --- | --- |
| **Ulceration** | **Erythema** |
| 0=no lesion | 0=none |
| 1=<1 cm$^2$ | 1=not severe |
| 2=1–3 cm$^2$ | 2=severe |
| 3=>3 cm$^2$ | |

**Figure 6.5 Oral Mucositis Assessment Scale.** Data from Sonis et al [6].

## The ideal mucositis scale

It would be very desirable to have a single scale to describe mucositis severity. At the moment there are well over a dozen different scoring instruments that are used, and having no consistent and universally used scale is a detriment when comparing regimen toxicities or evaluating new agents. Consequently, although a single scoring system would be ideal, it is probably a long way off. Figure 6.6 gives the key characteristics of the ideal mucositis scale.

## Variability between mucositis scales

Interestingly, the severity of mucositis is not evenly reflected across scales. What may be graded as severe in one scale may be slight or moderate in another. Some real examples will illustrate this point.

Two studies were conducted to describe the effect of a new antimucositis drug on the course of severe mucositis following the administration of a particular conditioning regimen prior to HSCT. Each study used a different scale to measure mucositis severity (Figure 6.7). In the first study,

**The ideal mucositis scale**

- Accurately reflects severity and course of objective and subjective clinical changes
- Easy to teach and use, with minimal inter-observer variability
- Does not require lesion measurement
- Sensitive enough to discriminate treatment efficacy
- Clinically meaningful
- Easily interpretable end points for clinicians, patients and FDA (labeling)

**Figure 6.6 The ideal mucositis scale.** Data from Treister et al [9].

| Effect of scale selection on study outcomes | | |
| --- | --- | --- |
| | **Active** | **Placebo** |
| Study 1 | 4.8 ± 4.7 days | 4.4 ± 2.7 days |
| Study 2 | 11.9 ± 6.1 days | 16.6 ± 8.9 days |

**Figure 6.7 Effect of scale selection on study outcomes.** This table presents the results of two studies in which GM-CSF was assessed for its efficacy in attenuating mucositis in HSCT patients. In Study 1 [10], mucositis was scored using NCI-CTC criteria, while mucositis severity was determined in the second study [11] using a more descriptive scoring scale. The differences in outcomes are dramatic. HSCT, hematopoietic stem cell transplant; GM-CSF, granulocyte macrophage colony-stimulating factor; NCI-CTC, National Cancer Institute Common Toxicity Criteria.

the duration of severe mucositis was the same among patients who received the test drug and those who received placebo [10]. In the second study, not only was the duration of mucositis in placebo patients almost four times that observed in the first study (16.6 days vs. 4.4 days), but the duration in patients being treated with the interventional drug was 11.9 days vs. 4.8 days in the first study [11]. Importantly, the *only* difference between the two studies was the scale used to measure mucositis.

In another study, mucositis was measured using two scales in the same patient population (Figure 6.8). Mucositis was scored using WHO or RTOG criteria. WHO grading is dependent on both objective (ulceration yes/no) and subjective (patients' ability to eat solids, liquids or nothing) variables. In contrast, RTOG grading is completely reliant on a clinician's ability to judge the size and characteristics of ulceration. In the example below, it is clear that incorporating patients' input into establishing the extent of ulceration markedly impacts scoring. Whereas 93% of patients graded by RTOG criteria were assigned a score of 2 (moderate mucositis), this characterization applied to only 51% of patients when WHO grading was used. Likewise, whereas 49% of subjects had severe mucositis by WHO criteria, the incidence was much smaller (7%) when RTOG criteria were used.

This illustrates very well the difference in how the description of stomatotoxicity would read. If RTOG criteria were used (similar to NCI-CTC), one would conclude that the risk of grade 3/4 mucositis was only 7% (for reasons that are unclear, reporting of toxicities is largely limited to grade 3/4 despite overwhelming evidence that the impact on patients for any toxicity is significant). In contrast, if WHO criteria were

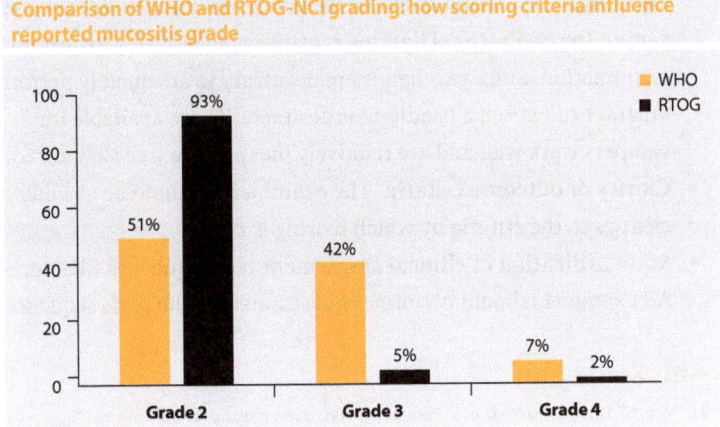

**Figure 6.8 Comparison of WHO and RTOG-NCI grading: how scoring criteria influence reported mucositis grade.** The severity of mucositis was graded using two scales in the same patients. The results of these evaluations, in over two hundred patients, would lead to very different conclusions about the stomatotoxicity of the regimen being tested. While one might conclude that the treatment was only mildly toxic based on NCI/RTOG criteria (only 7% of subjects developed severe [grade 3 or 4] mucositis), a completely different deduction might be made when WHO scores were seen and 49% of patients had severe mucositis.

the basis for a toxicity description, an entirely different conclusion – 49% of patients developed severe mucositis – would be reached.

## Minimizing inter-observer variability

A major challenge with any scale that depends on clinical judgment for its determination is the minimization of inter-observer variability. For the assessment of mucositis, a number of factors impact the accuracy of grading and differences in scoring of the same patient by different evaluators. These include the following:

- **Training.** In many instances, clinicians receive little or no formal training on how an oral examination is performed. Consequently the rigor of the evaluation may vary from one person who evaluates all mucosal sites in a systematic way to another who only looks at the dorsal surface of the tongue and palate. Aggressive training in the technique and scoring criteria will help minimize variability.

- **Lighting.** It is difficult to assess the condition of the mucosa if one cannot see easily. Good lighting is essential to assuring an accurate examination. Since two hands are necessary to adequately perform an oral evaluation, a headlight is desirable. Those available for campers work well and are relatively inexpensive (see Chapter 5).
- **Clarity of outcome criteria.** The examiner(s) should be absolutely clear as to the criteria by which scoring is done.
- **Standardization of clinical assessment technique** (see Chapter 5). All examiners should perform the assessment in the same sequence.

## References

1   Sonis ST, Elting LS, Keefe D, et al. Perspectives on cancer therapy-induced mucosal injury: pathogenesis, measurement, epidemiology, and consequences for patients. *Cancer*. 2004;100(suppl):1995-2025.
2   Eilers J, Berger AM, Petersen MC. Development, testing, and application of the oral assessment guide. *Oncol Nurs Forum*. 1988;15:325-330.
3   Dyck S. Development of a staging system for chemotherapy-induced stomatitis. Western Consortium for Cancer Nursing Research. *Cancer Nurs*. 1991;14:6-12.
4   Dibble SL, Shiba G, MacPhail L, Dodd MJ. MacDibbs Mouth Assessment. A new tool to evaluate mucositis in the radiation therapy patient. *Cancer Pract*. 1996;4:135-140.
5   Potting CM, Blijlevens NA, Donnelly JP, et al. A scoring system for the assessment of oral mucositis in daily nursing practice. *Eur J Cancer Care*. 2006;15:228-234.
6   Sonis ST, Eilers JP, Epstein JB, et al. Validation of a new scoring system for assessment of clinical trial research of oral mucositis induced by radiation or chemotherapy: Mucositis Study Group. *Cancer*. 1999;85:2103-2113.
7   McGuire DB, Peterson DE, Muller S, et al. The 20 item oral mucositis index: reliability and validity in bone marrow and stem cell transplant patients. *Cancer Invest*. 2002;20:893-903.
8   Tardieu C, Cowen D, Thirion X, Franquin JC. Quantitative scale of oral mucositis associated with autologous bone marrow transplantation. *Eur J Cancer B Oral Oncol*. 1996;32B:381-387.
9   Treister N, Sonis S. Oral mucositis. In: Ettinger DS, ed. *Supportive Care in Cancer Therapy*. Totowa, NJ: Humana Press; 2009:191-211.
10  Dazzi C, Cariello A, Giovanis P, et al. Prophylaxis with GM-CSF mouthwashes does not reduce frequency and duration of severe oral mucositis in patients with solid tumors undergoing high-dose chemotherapy with autologous peripheral blood stem cell transplantation rescue: a double blind, randomized, placebo-controlled study. *Ann Oncol*. 2003;14:559-563.
11  Bez C, Demarosi F, Sardella A, et al. GM-CSF mouthrinses in the treatment of severe oral mucositis: a pilot study. *Oral Surg Oral Med Oral Pathol Oral Radiol Endod*. 1999;88:311-315.

Development of this book was supported by funding from Helsinn

# Chapter 7

# Patient-reported outcomes

While we rely heavily on clinician evaluation of the mouth to define the course of mucositis, patient-reported outcomes (PROs) provide an important component to the overall assessment of the condition. PROs are especially significant because there is often a disconnect between how clinicians and patients view the severity of mucositis.

## Patient-reported outcome instruments for mucositis

There are a number of PRO instruments for mucositis. In general these tools rely on one of two types of scales to gather severity information: categorical scales and visual analog scales.

Categorical scales, for example the Oral Mucositis Daily Questionnaire, (OMDQ) (Figure 7.1) [1], ask patients to grade mucositis symptoms by circling a prescribed hierarchical list of possible outcomes. For example, they might ask the patient to circle a description of their mouth pain in which the options are delineated or to circle a numerical indicator.

Alternatively, visual analog scales (VAS) are less defined. Typically they present patients with a 10 cm line with descriptors of extremes at either end, such as no pain on one end and worse possible pain on the other. Patients are then asked to put a mark at that position on the line that best describes their symptoms.

S. T. Sonis, *Oral Mucositis*,
DOI: 10.1007/978-1-907673-46-7_7, © Springer Healthcare 2012

## Oral Mucositis Daily Questionnaire

**1. How would you rate your OVERALL HEALTH during the LAST 24 HOURS? (circle one number)**

| 0 | 1 | 2 | 3 | 4 | 5 | 6 | 7 | 8 | 9 | 10 |
|---|---|---|---|---|---|---|---|---|---|----|

| Worst possible | Halfway between worst possible and perfect health | Perfect health |
|---|---|---|

**2. During the LAST 24 HOURS, how much MOUTH AND THROAT SORENESS did you have? (circle one number)**

| No soreness | 0 | → | If you circled 0, please skip to question 5 |
|---|---|---|---|
| A little soreness | 1 | | |
| Moderate soreness | 2 | | |
| Quite a lot of soreness | 3 | | |
| Extreme soreness | 4 | | |

**3. During the LAST 24 HOURS, how much did MOUTH AND THROAT SORENESS limit you in each of the following activities? (circle one number)**

|  | Not limited | Limited a little | Limited some | Limited a lot | Unable to do |
|---|---|---|---|---|---|
| A. Swallowing | 0 | 1 | 2 | 3 | 4 |
| B. Drinking | 0 | 1 | 2 | 3 | 4 |
| C. Eating | 0 | 1 | 2 | 3 | 4 |
| D. Talking | 0 | 1 | 2 | 3 | 4 |
| E. Sleeping | 0 | 1 | 2 | 3 | 4 |

**4. On a scale of 1 to 10, how would you rate your OVERALL MOUTH AND THROAT SORENESS during the LAST 24 HOURS? (circle one number)**

| 0 | 1 | 2 | 3 | 4 | 5 | 6 | 7 | 8 | 9 | 10 |
|---|---|---|---|---|---|---|---|---|---|----|

| No soreness | Halfway between worst possible and perfect health | Worst possible |
|---|---|---|

**5. During the LAST 24 HOURS, how much DIARRHEA did you have? (circle one number)**

| No diarrhea | 0 | → | If you circled 0, STOP here |
|---|---|---|---|
| A little diarrhea | 1 | | |
| Moderate diarrhea | 2 | | |
| Quite a lot of diarrhea | 3 | | |
| Severe diarrhea | 4 | | |

**6. On a scale of 1 to 10, how would you rate your OVERALL DIARRHEA during the LAST 24 HOURS? (circle one number)**

| 0 | 1 | 2 | 3 | 4 | 5 | 6 | 7 | 8 | 9 | 10 |
|---|---|---|---|---|---|---|---|---|---|----|

| No diarrhea | Halfway between worst possible and perfect health | Worst possible diarrhea |
|---|---|---|

**Figure 7.1 Oral Mucositis Daily Questionnaire.** Reproduced with permission from Stiff et al [1].

# Categories of patient-reported outcomes

Generally PROs for mucositis fall into two categories based on their specificity. Some are mucositis-specific and seek patient input around symptoms and/or functional consequences related solely to mucositis. Among these are the OMDQ (Figure 7.1) [1], the OMAS (Figure 7.2) [2], the Patient-Reported Oral Mucositis Symptom (PROMS) scale (Figure 7.3) [3]. The second category is broader in scope insofar as these instruments

## Oral Mucositis Assessment Scale

**Radiation**

**Patient ID:**                                                    **Patient initials:**

**Patient diary date:**      /      /      (mm/dd/yy)  **Time:**   :      (24 hour clock)

### Mouth pain

Please indicate by a vertical line on the scale line below how severe the pain in your mouth is NOW

| 0 | 1 | 2 | 3 | 4 | 5 | 6 | 7 | 8 | 9 | 10 |
|---|---|---|---|---|---|---|---|---|---|---|

No pain                                                                              Most
                                                                                     severe pain

### Impact on swallowing:

Please indicate by a vertical line on the scale below how well you can swallow

| 0 | 1 | 2 | 3 | 4 | 5 | 6 | 7 | 8 | 9 | 10 |
|---|---|---|---|---|---|---|---|---|---|---|

No                                                                            Cannot swallow
trouble                                                                       anything at all
swallowing                                                                    (even saliva)

### Please indicate how well you can swallow foods or liquids by checking below:

**Function:**

Normal                  ☐

Only soft, solid foods  ☐

Only liquids            ☐

No foods or liquids     ☐

**For the investigator: If patient did not fill in diary, please explain why**

**I have reviewed this form:**      /      /      (mm/dd/yy)

**Investigator's signature:**

**Figure 7.2 Oral Mucositis Assessment Scale.** Patients completed this form on each evaluation day after standardized instructions from Investigator 1. Patients indicated their ability to function based on the eating ability at the bottom of the page. Identical forms were completed by patients receiving chemotherapy or radiation therapy. Reproduced with permission from Sonis et al [2].

## Patient-Reported Oral Mucositis Symptom scale

**This questionnaire asks you to evaluate some situation you may have experienced in the past week. All of the situations refer to the condition of your mouth. You can indicate the severity of the situation by placing a vertical mark along the lines below**

*First, we will use this type of line to rate temperature as an example*

**On a hot day in the middle of the summer, if we asked you to rate how warm it was today, you would probably mark the line as follows:**

not warm at all                                        extremely warm

**On a cool day in the fall, you might indicate:**

not warm at all                                        extremely warm

**On a cold day in the winter, you might indicate:**

not warm at all                                        extremely warm

*To practice: Please tell me how warm it is outside today by placing a mark on the line below*

not warm at all                                        extremely warm

*Now that you know how to use this scale, please indicate to what degree these situations have affected you in the past week*

**Mouth pain**

no pain                                                worst possible pain

**Difficulty speaking because of mouth sores**

no trouble speaking                                    worst possible pain

**Restriction of speech because of mouth sores**

no restriction of speech                               complete restriction of speech

**Difficulty eating hard foods (hard bread, potato chip, etc) because of mouth sores**

no trouble eating hard foods                           impossible to eat hard foods

**Difficulty eating soft foods (Jello, pudding, etc) because of mouth sores**

no trouble eating soft foods                           impossible to eat soft foods

**Restriction of eating because of mouth sores**

no restriction of eating                               complete restriction of eating

**Difficulty swallowing because of mouth sores**

not difficult to swallow                               impossible to swallow

**Change in taste**

no change in taste                                     complete change in taste

**Figure 7.3 Patient-Reported Oral Mucositis Symptom scale.** Reproduced with permission from Kushner et al [3].

include symptoms of mucositis as one component of the overall scale. These scales are largely disease-based (eg, head and neck cancer), and include the Functional Assessment of Cancer Therapy – Head and Neck (FACT-HN) [4], the MD Anderson symptom inventory-head and neck module [5], and the Vanderbilt Head and Neck Symptom Survey [6].

## Patient-reported outcomes in the pediatric population

Because PROs in pediatric populations present special challenges, child-specific scales have been proposed. The Children's International Mucositis Evaluation Scale (ChIMES) is one such instrument [7]. It is a categorical scale which, like others in this genre, relies heavily on the use of figures (happy faces), rather than words, to obtain patient input (Figure 7.4).

## References

1  Stiff PI, Emmanouilides C, Bensinger WI, et al. Palifermin reduced patient-reported mouth and throat soreness and improves patient functioning in the hematopoietic stem-cell transplantation setting. *J Clin Oncol*. 2006; 24: 5186-5193.

2  Sonis ST, Eilers JP, Epstein JB, et al. Validation of a new scoring system for assessment of clinical trial research of oral mucositis induced by radiation or chemotherapy: Mucositis Study Group. *Cancer*. 1999;85:2103-2113.

3  Kushner JA, Lawrence HP, Shoval I, et al. Development and validation of a Patient-Reported Oral Mucositis Symptom (PROMS) scale. *J Can Dent Assoc*. 2008; 74: 59.

4  List MA, D'Antonio LL, Cella DF, et al. The Performance Status Scale for Head and Neck Cancer Patients and the Functional Assessment of Cancer Therapy-Head and Neck scale: A study of utility and validity. *Cancer*. 1996; 77: 2294-2301.

5  Rosenthal DI, Mendoza TR, Chambers MS, et al. The M.D. Anderson symptom inventory-head and neck module, a patient-reported outcome instrument, accurately predicts the severity of radiation-induced mucositis. *Int J Radiat Oncol Biol Phys*. 2008;72:1355-1361.

6  Murphy BA, Dietrich MS, Wells N, et al. Reliability and validity of the Vanderbilt Head and Neck Symptom Survey: a tool to assess symptom burden in patients treated with chemoradiation. *Head Neck*. 2010;32:26-37.

7  Tomlinson D, Gibson F, Treister N, et al. Understandability, content validity, and overall acceptability of the Children's International Mucositis Evaluation Scale (ChIMES): child and parent reporting. *J Pediatr Hematol Oncol*. 2009;31:416-423.

Development of this book was supported by funding from Helsinn

## Children's International Mucositis Evaluation Scale (ChIMES)

### Pain

1. Which of these faces best describes how much pain you feel in your mouth or throat? Circle one

| 0 | 1 | 2 | 3 | 4 | 5 |
|---|---|---|---|---|---|
| No hurt | Hurts little bit | Hurts little more | Hurts even more | Hurts whole lot | Hurts worst |

### Function

2. Which of these faces shows how hard it is for you to swallow your saliva today because of mouth or throat pain? Circle one ☐ I can't tell

| 0 | 1 | 2 | 3 | 4 | 5 |
|---|---|---|---|---|---|
| Not hard | Little bit hard | Little more hard | Even harder | Very hard | Can't swallow |

3. Which of these faces shows how hard it is for you to eat today because of mouth or throat pain? Circle one ☐ I can't tell

| 0 | 1 | 2 | 3 | 4 | 5 |
|---|---|---|---|---|---|
| Not hard | Little bit hard | Little more hard | Even harder | Very hard | Can't swallow |

4. Which of these faces shows how hard it is to drink today because of mouth or throat pain? Circle one ☐ I can't tell

| 0 | 1 | 2 | 3 | 4 | 5 |
|---|---|---|---|---|---|
| Not hard | Little bit hard | Little more hard | Even harder | Very hard | Can't swallow |

### Pain

5. Have you taken any medicine for pain today? ☐ Yes ☐ No

   If yes, was pain in your mouth or throat the reason you needed pain medicine? ☐ Yes ☐ No

### Appearance

6. Please ask an adult to look in your mouth. Can he or she see any mouth sores in your mouth today? ☐ Yes ☐ No ☐ I can't tell

**Figure 7.4 Children's International Mucositis Evaluation Scale (ChIMES).** Reproduced with permission from Tomlinson et al [7].

# Chapter 8

# Nonmucositis mouth lesions in patients being treated for cancer

Patients receiving cancer treatment, especially myelosuppressive chemotherapy, are at risk of developing oral lesions exclusive of mucositis. The most common are those associated with opportunistic mucosal infections and, in the case of allogeneic HSCT recipients, oral lesions of graft-versus-host disease (GVHD). Lesion location, presentation and course are the key elements in making a correct diagnosis.

## Location

Mucositis is localized to the movable mucosa – the inner aspects of the lips, buccal mucosa, lateral and ventral surfaces of the tongue, floor of the mouth, soft palate and oropharynx. In contrast, opportunistic bacterial, viral and fungal infections often are located on the more keratinized tissues of the hard palate, dorsal tongue and gingiva. Similarly, oral GVHD typically manifests on both movable and nonmovable mucosa.

## Presentation

The clinical presentation of nonmucositis lesions varies, depending on etiology.

S. T. Sonis, *Oral Mucositis*,
DOI: 10.1007/978-1-907673-46-7_8, © Springer Healthcare 2012

## Bacterial infection

Oral bacterial infections in neutropenic patients often present as a necrotizing gingivitis characterized by necrosis of the papillary and marginal gingiva, a superficial pseudomembrane, and loss of typical gingival architecture (Figure 8.1).

## Viral infection

Oral manifestations of viral infections in myeloablated patients may vary from those typically described. Nonetheless, viral infections have a vesicular stage during which small clustering blisters are seen. Once the vesicles break, painful ulcerations develop. These differ from lesions of mucositis in that a pseudomembrane is not present and lesions are often located on the hard palate. Herpes viruses are most commonly implicated. Whereas the lesions of HSV tend to be bilateral, those of herpes zoster present in a unilateral vesicular pattern that is often linear [1] (Figure 8.2).

## Fungal infection

Candidiasis is the most common fungal infection in myeloablated cancer patients. Its frequency is also increased in patients in whom the normal oral environment is altered (ie, patients receiving chemoradiation therapy for cancers of the head and neck in which salivary function is disrupted). While the textbook description of oral candidiasis is one of necrotic, curdy, white clusters of organisms (pseudomembranous candidiasis), the infection may take different presentations, including areas

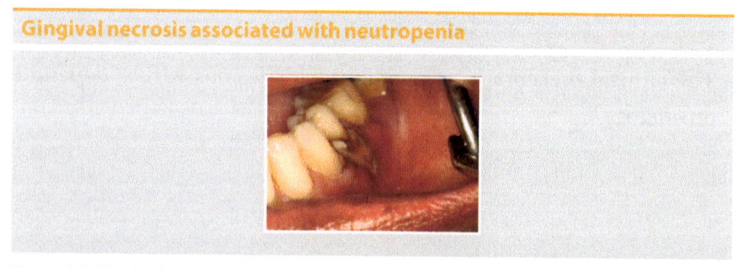

Gingival necrosis associated with neutropenia

**Figure 8.1 Gingival necrosis associated with neutropenia.** Gingival lesions that arise as a consequence of neutropenia (agranulocytosis) have a clinical presentation that is similar to acute necrotizing ulcerative gingivitis. Necrosis of the attached, marginal, and papillary gingiva and loss of papillary architecture are seen. A necrotic psuedomembrane is present and patients often complain of pain. © Nathaniel Treister, reproduced with permission.

of erythema, hyperplasia, or angular cheilitis (Figure 8.3). Because the latter occurs at the corners of the mouth, it is unlikely to be confused with a diagnosis of mucositis [2].

Deep fungal infections are a rare, but serious occurrence, which are noted most frequently in patients who undergo prolonged immunosuppression. Mucormycosis presents as a nonhealing invasive ulceration. Its appearance is similar to a tumor, and the diagnosis requires a biopsy [3].

**Herpes simplex infection**

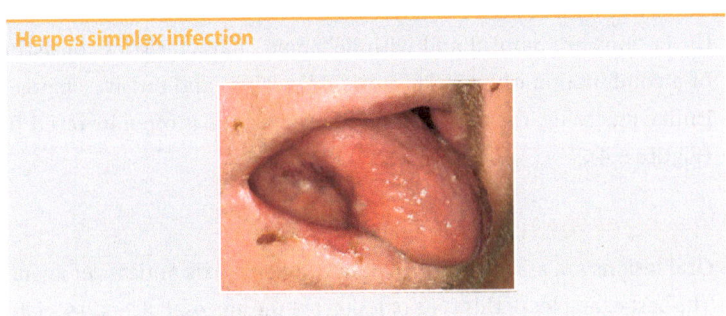

**Figure 8.2 Herpes simplex infection.** Among myeloablated cancer patients, oral viral infections are most often associated with organisms of the herpes group. Of these, herpes simplex 1 infections are the most common. While most often limited to extraoral vesicular lesions in healthy patients, they can occur intraorally in patients who are immuno- or myelosuppressed. © Nathaniel Treister, reproduced with permission.

**Candidiasis**

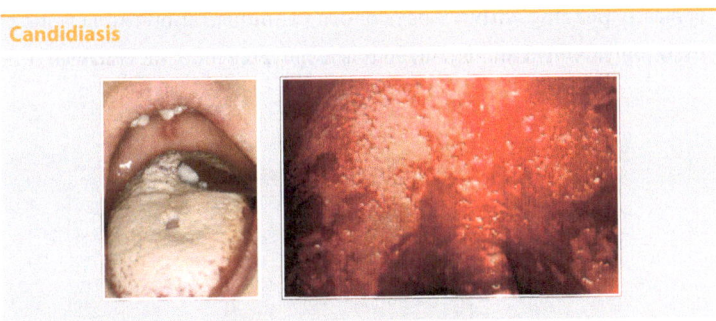

**Figure 8.3 Candidiasis.** *Candida albicans* is the most common cause of fungal infections in cancer patients. In addition to being neutropenic, changes in salivary volume and consistency often predispose to the development of thrush. While the classic lesion of candidiasis is described as a white, curdy, scrapable mass representing colonies of fungi, the condition may also present as uncomfortable areas of erythema (often of the palate) or angular cheilosis. © Nathaniel Treister, reproduced with permission.

## Graft-versus-host disease

GVHD is commonly manifested in the mouth. Since chronic GVHD occurs well after transplant (>100 days) [4] it is not a consideration in the differential diagnosis of mucositis. Acute GVHD may occur as soon as 3 weeks after transplant. In contrast, mucositis typically begins in closer proximity to the conditioning regimen, usually about 4 days later, peaks by 10 days and resolves in 3 to 4 weeks (Chapter 1). Thus, the patients' mucositis is typically resolved before the onset of GVHD.

The clinical appearance of oral GVHD differs from that of mucositis. Lesions are painful and with lichenoid characteristics consisting of a combination of hyperkeratotic, blistering, and erosive changes. Unlike mucositis, the dorsal surface of the tongue is often involved [5] (Figure 8.4).

## Atypical forms of mucositis

Oral lesions are associated with newer noncytotoxic anticancer agents. The best examples of this type of lesion are the mucosal ulcers associated with the administration of mammalian target of rapamycin (mTOR)-inhibitors [6,7]. This class of agents have been recently approved for the treatment of renal cell cancers, but may soon be available for other cancers. Ulcer onset is more acute than with conventional chemotherapy, typically peaking within 5 days of drug administration [8]. Lesions are extremely painful and localized to the movable mucosa. However, their

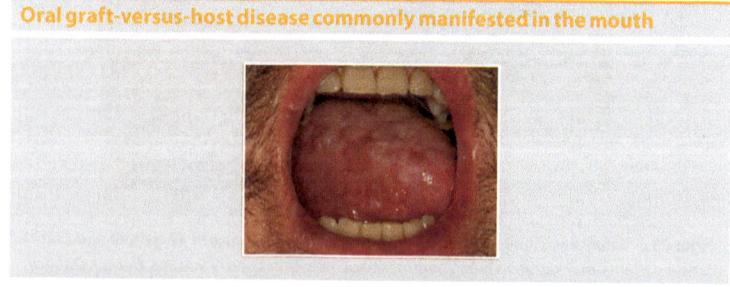

**Oral graft-versus-host disease commonly manifested in the mouth**

**Figure 8.4 Oral graft-versus-host disease commonly manifested in the mouth.** Lesions present as lichenoid areas associated with erosive or ulcerative changes. Like mucositis, these lesions are painful and often modify patients' ability to eat. Unlike mucositis, they are limited to recipients of allogeneic HSCT and typically begin at least 4 weeks following transplant. HSCT, hematopoietic stem cell transplant. © Nathaniel Treister, reproduced with permission.

clinical appearance is analogous to that noted for aphthous stomatitis and consists of oval ulcers with a grayish necrotic center surrounded by an erythematous periphery [8] (Figure 8.5).

### mTOR-inhibitor-associated stomatitis (mIAS)

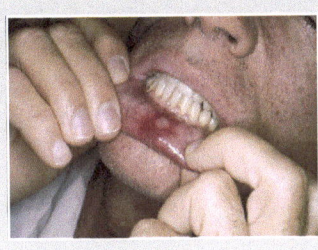

**Figure 8.5 mTOR-inhibitor-associated stomatitis (mIAS).** Oral mucosal ulcerations associated with the administration of mTOR-inhibitors are illustrative of the diversity of mucosal toxicities associated with new classes of anticancer agents. mIAS has been consistently reported to occur in at least 40% of patients treated with this form of therapy. Unlike ulcers associated with mucositis caused by cytotoxic agents, mIAS lesions begin shortly after drug administration and present as round ulcers with a grayish necrotic center and surrounded by an erythematous border. Clinically the lesions are indistinguishable from those associated with aphthous stomatitis. © Nathaniel Treister, reproduced with permission.

## References

1 Sciubba JJ. Oral mucosal diseases in the office setting – Part 1: Aphthous stomatitis and herpes simplex infections. *Gen Dent*. 2007;55:347-354.
2 Sherman RG, Prusinski L, Ravenel MC, Joralmon RA. Oral candidosis. *Quintessence Int*. 2002;33:521-532.
3 Scully C, de Almeida OP. Orofacial manifestations of the systemic mycoses. *J Oral Pathol Med*. 1992;21:289-294.
4 Horwitz ME, Sullivan KM. Chronic graft-versus-host disease. *Blood Rev*. 2006; 20: 15-27.
5 Imanguli MM, Alevizos I, Brown R, et al. Oral graft-versus-host disease. *Oral Dis*. 2008;14:396-412.
6 Raymond E, Alexandre J, Faivre S, et al. Safety and pharmacokinetics of escalated doses of weekly intravenous infusion of CCI-779, a novel mTOR inhibitor, in patients with cancer. *J Clin Oncol*. 2004;22:2336-2347.
7 Sonis S, Treister N, Chawla S, et al. Preliminary characterization of oral lesions associated with inhibitors of mammalian target of rapamycin in cancer patients. *Cancer*. 2010;116:210-215.
8 Sankhala K, Mita A, Kelly K, et al. The emerging safety profile of mTOR inhibitors, a novel class of anticancer agents. *Target Oncol*. 2009;4:135-142.

Development of this book was supported by funding from Helsinn

# Chapter 9

# Current approaches to the management of oral mucositis

Despite its frequency, impact on patients and health and economic costs, there are currently limited evidence-based options for the prevention or treatment of OM. A number of guidelines for the management of OM have been thoughtfully prepared by the Multinational Association of Supportive Care in Cancer (MASCC) [1], the American Society of Clinical Oncology (ASCO) [2], and the National Comprehensive Cancer Network (NCCN) panels [3]. For the most part, they are in agreement. This chapter attempts to summarize the current standard of care for mucositis management in a way that presents a consensus of current recommendations.

## Optimization of oral health

Good oral health appears to be an advantage in reducing the risk, severity, and course of OM [4]. Optimization of oral health begins with a thorough examination of the mouth and dentition prior to the start of cancer therapy in order to identify pre-existing disease or sources of mucosal irritation. For example, patients with poorly fitting dentures or orthodontic appliances may have incipient mucosal injury that exacerbates the impact of stomatotoxic therapy [5]. Consequently, orthodontic bands should be removed prior to chemotherapy. Patients with oral prosthesis should be advised to leave them out as much as possible [6]. Poorly fitting appliances should be adjusted. Sharp or fractured teeth should be restored, smoothed or removed.

S. T. Sonis, *Oral Mucositis*,
DOI: 10.1007/978-1-907673-46-7_9, © Springer Healthcare 2012

The mouth harbors a large numbers of microorganisms, many of which colonize the teeth and mucosa. While mucositis is not an infectious disease, secondary colonization of ulcerated areas likely retards healing. Importantly, in myeloablated patients ulcerated mucosa can act as a portal for systemic entry of organisms. Consequently, a reduction in the oral bacterial load through aggressive oral hygiene is viewed positively. Since many treatment regimens may adversely affect salivary flow, patients' ability to physiologically clear oral organisms can be retarded.

### The importance of patient education

Patients should be educated on the value of good oral health relative to the cancer therapy. Oral hygiene instruction should be given, which includes toothbrushing, flossing, and rinsing with bland (saline or sodium bicarbonate) solutions. There are data to support the notion that this may be best accomplished through the use of a multidisciplinary team that couples nurses and dental professionals [1]. It is also helpful to provide regular feedback to patients on the effectiveness of their oral hygiene efforts. Regular oral assessment during therapy is therefore an important component of a program to assure maximum oral health.

## The role of diet

Diet plays a role in oral health. Therefore, patients should be advised on food selections that promote, or which could interfere with, oral health. Since patients may experience modification of taste, changes in appetite, and dysphagia, food recommendations need to balance the need to maintain intake with the increased risk of oral disease. Avoidance of foods containing processed sugar, particularly those of a sticky consistency, should be discussed. Acidic and spicy foods may exacerbate the discomfort of mucositis and should be avoided. Common sense and patient tolerance are excellent guides to food selection with respect to consistency, texture, and flavoring.

## Cryotherapy

The use of oral cryotherapy (ice chips) for the management of mucositis has been suggested for quite some time [7]. Although the optimal time for which patients need to hold ice chips in their mouths around the time of their chemotherapy has been the debated and studied, it appears that a 30 to 60 minute exposure period may be helpful. The lack of expense or toxicity and relative ease of use make this form of treatment something to be considered for chemotherapeutic agents which have a short half-life.

## Biologicals and drugs

### Palifermin

Palifermin (keratinocyte growth factor-1) is the only biological or pharmacological agent approved for an OM indication in the US. Its use is restricted to mucositis associated with conditioning regimens administered in preparation for HSCT in patients being treated for hematological malignancies [3]. Results of a pivotal Phase 3 study in which the agent was compared to placebo in 212 patients demonstrated a significant reduction in the duration and severity of OM in patients treated with palifermin compared to placebo. Quality of life outcomes were also favorably affected [8]. Palifermin is administered intravenously for 3 days prior to the start of chemotherapy and for an additional 3 days beginning on the day of transplant [3].

### Benzydamine HCl

Benzydamine HCl has been deemed safe and effective in patients being treated for cancers of the head and neck with radiation therapy only as described in the MASCC guidelines [1], but not with the more standard concomitant chemotherapy/radiation regimens. It is approved for use in Europe, Canada, and Australia as well as in some countries in South America and Asia, but not in the US. In those areas where it has been approved, it represents a potential intervention for a limited number of patients.

### Amifostine

Amifostine is a free-radical scavenger that has been approved in a number of countries worldwide (including the US and across the EU) for the prevention of radiation-induced xerostomia in patients receiving radiation therapy for the treatment of cancers of the head and neck [3]. It has been suggested that it may have efficacy in the management of mucositis, based on its utility in treating radiation-induced esophagitis [9]. However, clinical data to support its use in the treatment of OM is lacking [10].

## Palliative preparations

### Magic mouthwashes

Magic mouthwashes refer to a collection of formulations that are largely institution specific. Many have been created around institutional folk-lore. Although the specific components of magic mouthwashes vary, in general each contains a topical anesthetic (lidocaine or Benadryl) in some coating agent (eg, Kaopectate, Milk of Magnesia). Additionally, depending on the institution, some contain an antifungal and/or an antibiotic, while others have a topical steroid added. Studies in which magic mouthwashes have been compared to standard of care rinses such as saline have consistently failed to demonstrate a benefit that would support the use of magic mouthwashes in OM [1,3].

## Medical devices for oral mucositis

There has been a proliferation in the number of devices that are available for the management of OM. In general, there is currently insufficient data to support the routine use of any of these products [3], as they are not subject to the same rigor of clinical testing that is required for drugs or biologicals. Devices fall into two main categories: adhesive gels, liquids, and dissolving tablets that coat injured mucosa to provide a barrier, and electrolyte solutions that were originally developed for treatment of the consequences of xerostomia.

### Coating formulations

Gelclair, MuGard, Mucotrol, and Episil are unique formulations of different coating agents used to palliate ulcerated mucosa. Gelclair is dispensed as a solution that, when mixed with a small volume of water, forms a viscous bioadhesive oral gel. Episil and MuGard are formulated as ready to use flowing gels or liquids that form a bioadhesive film when rinsed in the mouth. Mucotrol is available as a wafer, which when dissolved in mouth, coats the mucosa. Episil is only available in Europe whereas Gelclair, MuGuard, and Mucotrol are also available in the US.

Results of open-label studies suggest that Gelclair may enhance mucositis-related symptom control. Overall, 459 patients with oral complications have been treated with Gelclair in a total of 15 studies [11–23].

Similar efficacy conclusions were reached in a heterogeneous patient population (n=129) treated with MuGard for the prevention or treatment of mucosal injury associated with cytotoxic cancer therapy or other mucosal conditions [26].

The only data identified through a similar search for Mucotrol reported the results of a pilot study performed at a single institution, in which Mucotrol was compared to placebo [27]. This double-blind randomized trial enrolled 11 subjects to each study arm, but concluded that Mucotrol was of benefit in the treatment of mucositis associated with chemoradiation. A search of PubMed failed to identify publications of clinical studies.

Statistically powered, multi-center, prospective, randomized, placebo-controlled trials in which the efficacy of coating formulations are tested are not available and should be strongly encouraged to definitively evaluate the true value of these agents in managing mucositis.

## Electrolyte solutions

Two electrolyte solutions have been developed for use in patients with OM: Caphosol and NeutraSal. Caphosol is an artificial saliva comprised of neutral supersaturated calcium phosphate mouthrinse [28]. It is supplied in two solution containers that are reconstituted immediately prior to use. NeutraSal is an electrolyte solution of sodium bicarbonate and calcium and phosphate ions that is supplied as a powder that is reconstituted prior to use. As with the other devices, adequately powered, prospective trials are lacking. What data is available is inconsistent; one study of 95 patients [29] showed that calcium phosphate mouth rinse + fluoride significantly decreased duration of mucositis versus fluoride alone (3.72 days vs 7.22 days, $P=0.001$), whereas another study of 59 patients [30] did not find a significant difference in the development and severity of oral mucositis between patients receiving calcium phosphate mouth rinse and those receiving standard oral care. Prospectively randomized, blinded trials are needed to better understand the value of these agents as an intervention for OM compared with current oral care maintenance.

## The future

For the overwhelming majority of cancer patients, the prevention and management of OM remains a significant unmet clinical need. For healthcare professionals, OM is one of the most frustrating, treatment-altering side effects of cancer treatment. And for hospitals, clinics, and health insurers, mucositis results in significant drains of resources and funding [31].

Fortunately, with a better understanding of its pathobiology serving as a basis, a wide range of mechanistically-based therapies are in the development pipeline.

## References

1 Keefe DM, Schubert MM, Elting LS, et al. Updated clinical practice guidelines for the prevention and treatment of mucositis. *Cancer*. 2007;109:820-831.

2 Hensley ML, Hagerty KL, Kewalramani T, et al. American Society of Clinical Oncology 2008 clinical practice guideline update: Use of chemotherapy and radiation therapy protectants. *J Clin Oncol*. 2009;27:127-145.

3 Bensinger W, Schubert M, Ang KK, et al. NCCN Task Force Report: Prevention and management of mucositis in cancer care. *J Natl Compr Canc Netw*. 2008;6(suppl 1):S1-S21.

4 Djuric M, Hillier-Kolarov V, Belic A, Jankovic L. Mucositis prevention by improved dental care in acute leukemia patients. *Support Care Cancer*. 2006;14:137-146.

5 Schubert MM, Peterson DE, Lloid ME: Oral complications. In: Thomas ED, Blume KG, Forman SJ, eds. *Hematopoietic Cell Transplantation*, 2nd edn. Malden, MA: Blackwell Science Inc; 1999:751-763.

6 Scully C, Epstein J, Sonis S. Oral mucositis: a challenging complication of radiotherapy, chemotherapy, and radiochemotherapy. Part 2: diagnosis and management of mucositis. *Head Neck*. 2004;26:77-84.

7 Treister N, Sonis S. Oral mucositis. In: Ettinger DS, ed. *Cancer and Drug Discovery Development: Supportive Care in Cancer Therapy*. Totowa, NJ: Humana Press. 2008;193-211.

8 Spielberger R, Stiff P, Bensinger W, et al. Palifermin for oral mucositis after intensive therapy for hematologic cancers. *N Engl J Med*. 2004;351:2590-2598

9 Wynn RB, Mehta V. Reduction of treatment breaks and radiation-induced esophagitis and pneumonitis using amifostine in unresectable non-small cell lung cancer patients receiving definitive concurrent chemotherapy and radiation therapy: a prospective community-based clinical trial. *Sem Oncol*. 2005;32(2 suppl 3):S99-104.

10 Bensadoun RJ, Schubert MM, Lalla RV, Keefe D. Amifostine in the management of radiation-induced and chemo-induced mucositis. *Support Care Cancer*. 2006;14:566-572.

11 Flook C, Calman F, Mant M, et al. GELCLAIR® vs benzydamine in a randomised controlled study in patients with oral mucositis due to radical radiotherapy. *Support Care Cancer*. 2005;13:443-444.

12 McKenzie M, Papish S, Hansen V, et al. A randomized open label trial comparing Gelclair with institutional standard magic mouthwash for the treatment of pain associated with radiation or chemotherapy induced mucositis. *Support Cancer Care*. 2006;14:641.

13 Short L, Fung D. Clinical effectiveness of Gelclair in the treatment of oral mucositis: a patient based questionnaire. *Int J Paediatr Dent*. 2008;18(suppl 1):14.

14 Liewer SE, Hecht KA, Smith CF, et al. Gelclair® for the treatment of chemotherapy-induced stomatitis in transplant and hematology patients: an interim analysis. *Blood*. 2004;104: Abstract 5317.

15  De Cordi D, D'Andrea N, Giorgiutti A, Martina S. Gelclair: potentially an efficacious treatment for chemotherapy-induced mucositis. Presented at: Italian Anti-tumour League III Congress for Professional Oncology Nurses; October 10-12, 2001; Conegliano, Italy.

16  D'Andrea N, Giorgiutti E, De Cordi D, Piga A. Oral pharyngeal mucositis: Nursing assessment on the efficacy of a new treatment. *Ann Oncol*. 2003;14(suppl 4):iv97.

17  Bonassi L, Cotroneo G, Nastasi G. Treatment with gelclair in patients suffering grade III-IV oral mcositis: Efficacy and impact on quality of life (QOL). *Ann Oncol*. 2003;14(suppl 4):E38.

18  Lindsay G, Rushton R, Harris T, et al. The clinical effectiveness of Gelclair in the management of oral mucositis. *Austral Nurs J*. 2009;16:30-33.

19  Innocenti M, Moscatelli G, Lopez S. Efficacy of Gelclair in reducing pain in patients with oral lesions: Preliminary findings from an open pilot study. *J Pain Symptom Manage*. 2002;24:456-457.

20  Hita-Iglesias P, Torres-Lagares D, Gutiérrez-Pérez JL. Evaluation of the clinical behaviour of a polyvinylpyrrolidone and sodium hyalonurate gel (Gelclair) in patients subjected to surgical treatment with CO2 laser. *Int J Oral Maxillofac Surg*. 2006;35:514-517.

21  Berndtson M. A preliminary study of Orassist (Gelclair) in the management of oral mucositis. *Swedish Hospital Dentistry*. 2001;26:17-21.

22  Barber C, Powell R, Ellis A, Hewett J. Comparing pain control and ability to eat and drink with standard therapy vs Gelclair: a preliminary, double centre, randomised controlled trial on patients with radiotherapy-induced oral mucositis. *Support Care Cancer*. 2007;15:427-440.

23  McLean M. An Audit of the Efficacy of Gelclair® for Mouth Pain in Patients Undergoing Radiotherapy or Chemotherapy. Presented as a poster at 2009 BAHNON congress, UK.

24  Gibson F, Donachie PHJ, Blandford E, et al. Efficacy of Gelclair in reducing the pain of oral mucositis. Presented at the 42nd Congress of the International Society of Paediatric Oncology, October 21-24th, 2010, Boston, Massachusetts, USA.

25  Wildfang I, Tschechne B, Borghardt J, et al. Oropharyngeal mucositis prophylaxis in combined radioimmunochemotherapy. *J Clin Oncol*. 2010; 28 (suppl): Abstract e19613.

26  Duckert A, et al. Management of oral mucositis (OM) with a muco-adhesive oral rinse: European clinical experience. Abstract presented at the European Society for Medical Oncology Congress, Milan, 8-12 October 2010.

27  Naidu M, Ramana GV, Ratnam, SV et al. A randomized, double-blind, parallel, placebo-controlled study to evaluate the efficacy of MF5232 (Mucotrol), a concentrated oral gel wafer, in the treatment of oral mucositis. *Drugs RD*. 2005;6:291-298.

28  Abraham J. Calcium phosphate mouth rinse for preventing oral mucositis. *Commun Oncol*. 2008;5:171-172.

29  Papas AS, Clark RE, Martuscelli G, et al. A prospective, randomized trial for the prevention of mucositis in patients undergoing hematopoietic stem cell transplantation. *Bone Marrow Transplant*. 2003;31:705-712.

30  Stokman M, Burlage F, Spijkervet F, et al. The effect of a calcium phosphate mouth rinse on chemo/radiation induced oral mucositis in head and neck cancer patients. *Support Care Cancer*. 2010;S3:S114.

31  Elting LS, Cooksley CD, Chambers MS, Garden AS. Risk, outcomes, and costs of radiation-induced oral mucositis among patients with head-and-neck malignancies. *Int J Radiat Oncol Biol Phys*. 2007;68:1110-1120.

Development of this book was supported by funding from Helsinn

# Further reading

Barasch A, Peterson DE. Risk factors for ulcerative oral mucositis in cancer patients: unanswered questions. *Oral Oncol*. 2003;39:91-100.

Bensinger W, Schubert M, Ang KK, et al. NCCN Task Force Report: Prevention and management of mucositis in cancer care. *J Natl Compr Canc Netw*. 2008;6(suppl 1):S1-S21.

Bogunia-Kubik K. Polymorphisms within genes encoding TNF-alpha and TNF-beta associate with the incidence of post-transplant complications in recipients of allogeneic hematopoietic stem cell transplants. *Arch Immunol Ther Exp (Warsz)*. 2004; 52:240-249.

Cella D, Pulliam J, Fuchs H, et al. Evaluation of pain associated with oral mucositis during the acute period after administration of high-dose chemotherapy. *Cancer*. 2003;98:406-412.

Clarkson JE, Worthington HV, Furness S, et al. Interventions for treating oral mucositis for patients with cancer receiving treatment. *Cochrane Database Syst Rev*. 2010;8:CD001973.

Elting LS, Keefe DM, Sonis ST, et al. Patient-reported measurements of oral mucositis in head and neck cancer patients treated with radiotherapy with or without chemotherapy: demonstration of increased frequency, severity, resistance to palliation, and impact on quality of life. *Cancer*. 2008;113:2704-2713.

Etiz D, Orhan B, Demirüstü C, et al. Comparison of radiation-induced oral mucositis scoring systems. *Tumori*. 2002;88:379-384.

Hahn T, Zhelnova E, Sucheston L, et al. A deletion polymorphism in glutathione-S-transferase mu (GSTM1) and/or theta (GSTT1) is associated with an increased risk of toxicity after autologous blood and marrow transplantation. *Biol Blood Marrow Transplant*. 2010;16:801-808.

Imanguli MM. Alevizos I, Brown R, et al. Oral graft-versus-host disease. *Oral Dis*. 2008;14:396-412.

Jaroneski LA. The importance of assessment rating scales for chemotherapy-induced oral mucositis. *Oncol Nurs Forum*. 2006;33:1085-1090.

Keefe DM, Schubert MM, Elting LS, et al. Updated clinical practice guidelines for the prevention and treatment of mucositis. *Cancer*. 2007;109:820-831.

Lalla RV, Sonis ST, Peterson DE. Management of oral mucositis in patients who have cancer. *Dent Clin North Am*. 2008;52:61-77.

Lerman MA, Laudenbach J, Marty FM, et al. Management of oral infections in cancer patients. *Dent Clin North Am*. 2008;52:129-154.

McGuire DB, Peterson DE, Muller S, et al. The 20 item Oral Mucositis Index: reliability and validity in bone marrow and stem cell transplant patients. *Cancer Invest*. 2002;20:893-903.

Murphy BA. Clinical and economic consequences of mucositis induced by chemotherapy and/or radiation therapy. *J Support Oncol*. 2007;5(9 suppl 4):13-21.

Nonzee NJ, Dandade NA, Patel U, et al. Evaluating the supportive care costs of severe radiochemotherapy-induced mucositis and pharyngitis: results from a Northwestern University Costs of Cancer Program pilot study with head and neck and nonsmall cell lung cancer patients who received care at a county hospital, a Veterans Administration hospital, or a comprehensive cancer care center. *Cancer*. 2008;113:1446-1452.

Peterson DE, Bensadoun RJ, Roila F, ESMO Guidelines Working Group. Management of oral and gastrointestinal mucositis: ESMO clinical recommendations. *Ann Oncol*. 2009;20(Suppl 4):174-177.

Potting CM, Blijlevens NA, Donnelly JP, et al. A scoring system for the assessment of oral mucositis in daily nursing practice. *Eur J Cancer Care*. 2006;15:228-234.

S. T. Sonis, *Oral Mucositis*,
DOI: 10.1007/978-1-907673-46-7, © Springer Healthcare 2012

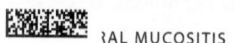 

Scully C, Epstein J, Sonis S. Oral mucositis: a challenging complication of radiotherapy, chemotherapy and radiochemotherapy. Part 2: diagnosis and management of mucositis. *Head Neck.* 2004;26:77-84.

Scully C, Sonis S, Diz PD. Oral mucositis. *Oral Dis.* 2006;12:229-241.

Sonis ST. Mucositis as a biological process: a new hypothesis for the development of chemotherapy-induced stomatotoxicity. *Oral Oncol.* 1998;34:39-43.

Sonis ST. A biological approach to mucositis. *J Support Oncol.* 2004;2:21-32.

Sonis ST. Pathobiology of oral mucositis: novel insights and opportunities. *J Support Oncol.* 2007;5(9 suppl 4):3-11.

Sonis ST. Mucositis: The impact, biology and therapeutic opportunities of oral mucositis. *Oral Oncol.* 2009;45:1015-1020.

Sonis ST. New thoughts on the initiation of mucositis. *Oral Dis.* 2010;16:597-600.

Sonis ST, Eilers JP, Epstein JB, et al. Validation of a new scoring system for the assessment of clinical trial research of oral mucositis induced by radiation or chemotherapy. *Cancer.* 1999;85:2103-2113.

Sonis ST, Elting LS, Keefe D, et al. Perspectives on cancer therapy-induced mucosal injury: pathogenesis, measurement, epidemiology, and consequences for patients. *Cancer.* 2004;100(9 suppl):1995-2025.

Sonis ST, Oster G, Fuchs H, et al. Oral mucositis and the clinical and economic outcomes of hematopoietic stem-cell transplantation. *J Clin Oncol.* 2001;19:2201-2205.

Sonis S, Treister N, Chawla S, et al. Preliminary characterization of oral lesions associated with inhibitors of mammalian target of rapamycin in cancer patients. *Cancer.* 2010;116:210-215.

Stokman MA, Sonis ST, Dijkstra PU, et al. Assessment of oral mucositis in clinical trials: impact of training on evaluators in a multi-centre trial. *Eur J Cancer.* 2005;41:1735-1738.

Sung L, Tomlinson GA, Greenberg ML, et al. Validation of the Oral Mucositis Assessment Scale in pediatric cancer. *Pediatr Blood Cancer.* 2007;49:149-153.

Vera-Llonch M, Oster G, Hagiwara M, et al. Oral mucositis in patients undergoing treatment for head and neck carcinoma. *Cancer.* 2006;106:329-336.

Woo SB, Sonis ST, Sonis AL. The role of herpes simplex virus in the development of oral mucositis in bone marrow transplant recipients. *Cancer.* 1990; 66:2375-2379.

Worthington HV, Clarkson JE, Khalid T, et al. Interventions for treating oral candidiasis for patients with cancer receiving treatment. *Cochrane Database Syst Rev.* 2010;7:CD001972.